DIGESTIVE DISEASES - RESEARCH AND CLINICAL DEVELOPMENTS

SHORT BOWEL SYNDROME (SBS)

SYMPTOMS, SURGICAL OUTCOMES AND COMPLICATIONS

Digestive Diseases - Research and Clinical Developments

Additional books in this series can be found on Nova's website under the Series tab.

Additional e-books in this series can be found on Nova's website under the eBooks tab.

DIGESTIVE DISEASES - RESEARCH AND CLINICAL DEVELOPMENTS

SHORT BOWEL SYNDROME (SBS)

SYMPTOMS, SURGICAL OUTCOMES AND COMPLICATIONS

VIOLET CHAPMAN
EDITOR

NOVA BIOMEDICAL
New York

Library of Congress Cataloging-in-Publication Data

Library of Congress Control Number: 2016933876

ISBN: 978-1-63484-944-9

Published by Nova Science Publishers, Inc. † New York

CONTENTS

PREFACE

Short bowel syndrome (SBS) is a pathologic condition which is characterized by reduced intestinal length and diminished intestinal absorptive capacity mainly due to extensive surgical resection, congenital defect, or pathological process affecting the small bowel. In recent decades, a better understanding of the underlying pathophysiology, new and modified surgical techniques and improvements in enteral and parenteral nutritional support improved the results of therapy of patients with SBS. This book provides research on the etiology, symptoms, surgical options and outcomes, and complications of SBS.

Chapter 1 - Adequate nutrition necessitates a normal length and normal function (digestive and absorptive) of the small bowel mucosa. Malnutrition occurs when any of the above factors is diminished beyond a crucial point. Surgical resection of approximately half of the small bowel significantly impairs intestinal absorption; resection of more than 70% of the small bowel is associated with significant mortality. In recent decades, a better understanding of the underlying pathophysiology, new and modified surgical techniques and improvements in enteral and parenteral nutritional support improved the results of therapy of patients with short bowel syndrome (SBS). The term intestinal failure (IF) is rather depicting the functional aspect of the SBS and is independent of its length; in these cases the length may be adequate but the small bowel doesn't meet the body's requirements in nutrients. The aim of initial surgical therapy is the salvage of small bowel to prevent the development of SBS and to achieve the maintenance of fluid and electrolyte balance. In selected patients with rapid intestinal transit and dilated bowel, longitudinal intestinal lengthening and tailoring (LILT) and serial transverse enteroplasty (STEP) may provide some benefit. Clinical outcomes indicate similar results for both STEP and LILT procedures. In the absence of bowel dilation, segmental reversal of the small bowel may reduce parenteral nutrition (PN) requirements. Intestinal transplantation is the last option in cases where all previous surgical attempts have failed and where life-threatening complications of PN have occurred. The results of small bowel transplantation - once being disappointing because of the high rate of rejection - seem nowadays to be promising partially due to the improvements in immunosuppressive therapy (using alemtuzumab). Multivisceral transplantation, for multi-organ involvement (liver/small bowel) is performed in very few centers worldwide; more studies are needed to confirm the benefit of multivisceral transplantation for patients with SBS. Therapeutic manipulations towards the growth of tissue-engineered small intestine using stem cells and biopharmaceuticals are emerging therapeutic approaches, developed during the past decade; the effectiveness of these therapeutic strategies remains unproven.

Chapter 2 - Short bowel syndrome (SBS) refers to the malabsorptive state caused by physical and functional loss of portions of the small intestine, most frequently following extensive intestinal resection. Following resection, intestinal tissue undergoes morphological and functional changes to compensate for the losts function of the resected bowel, and extent of adaptation depends on resected bowel anatomy and the amount of remaining bowel. The clinical symptoms associated with SBS vary according to the length and location of the affected small bowel, the presence and nature of the underlying disease, and the presence or absence of the large bowel and ileocecal valve. The goals of medical treatment are to maintain fluid, electrolyte, and nutrient balances, as well as appropriate disease management to advoid side effects. In the past, all patients were managed on total parenteral nutrition at home. The development of medical therapies, such as recombinant growth hormone, octreotide and glucagon-like-peptide-2 analogs, has helped increases the intestinal absorption capacity. There are several surgical options to manage SBS. Technique choice depends on the patient´s underlying pathophysiology, and includes factors like intestinal transit time, remnant bowel length, presence of an intact colon, and degree of small bowel dilatation. Intestinal transplantation has been increasingly used with improving success in patients with intestinal failure life-threatening complications. The author's should continue to emphasize prevention of intestinal resection and conservation of as much intestine as possible in massive resection.

Chapter 3 - Intestinal failure (IF) in the pediatric population most commonly results from a congenital abnormality or major intra-abdominal catastrophe in the neonatal period or early in life. The term short bowel syndrome (SBS) is commonly used interchangeably with IF and is one of the most common causes of pediatric IF although other etiologies of IF exist despite normal or near normal bowel length. The management of both IF and SBS currently relies upon parenteral nutrition (PN), but the surgical management of SBS has undergone an extensive maturation process in the last several decades. While intestinal transplantation is now a viable option for some patients, it is still far from first line therapy and outcomes have lagged behind those of other organs. The central tenet of the currently available and emerging surgical intestinal lengthening techniques is increasing the function and absorptive capacity of the remaining bowel. As early as the late 19th century, animal models were used to develop viable lengthening procedures, which led to innovative procedures of the time including antiperistaltic segments, valves and intestinal pacing. These early developments spurred the evolution of techniques as surgical intervention proved effective in increasing intestinal function. More recently, the serial transverse enteroplasty (STEP) and spiral intestinal lengthening and tailoring (SILT) procedures have been developed, taking advantage of progress in understanding of bowel physiology and decades of surgical experience. This review will summarize the current state of surgical approaches to bowel lengthening, with a brief overview of pertinent historical procedures important in the progression of management of this disease.

In: Short Bowel Syndrome (SBS)
Editor: Violet Chapman
ISBN: 978-1-63484-944-9

Chapter 1

SHORT BOWEL SYNDROME (SBS): SYMPTOMS, SURGICAL OUTCOMES AND COMPLICATIONS

Dimitrios K. Nasikas, MD,
and George H. Sakorafas*, MD, PhD
Department of Surgical Oncology,
Saint Savvas Cancer Hospital, Athens, Greece

ABSTRACT

Adequate nutrition necessitates a normal length and normal function (digestive and absorptive) of the small bowel mucosa. Malnutrition occurs when any of the above factors is diminished beyond a crucial point. Surgical resection of approximately half of the small bowel significantly impairs intestinal absorption; resection of more than 70% of the small bowel is associated with significant mortality. In recent decades, a better understanding of the underlying pathophysiology, new and modified surgical techniques and improvements in enteral and parenteral nutritional support improved the results of therapy of patients with short bowel syndrome (SBS). The term intestinal failure (IF) is rather depicting the functional aspect of the SBS and is independent of its

* Address for the correspondence: George H. Sakorafas, MD, PhD, Chairman, Department of Surgical Oncology, Saint Savvas Cancer Hospital, Arkadias 19-21, 115 26 Athens, Greece, Tel/Fax+ 30 2107487192, email: georgesakorafas@yahoo.com.

length; in these cases the length may be adequate but the small bowel doesn't meet the body's requirements in nutrients. The aim of initial surgical therapy is the salvage of small bowel to prevent the development of SBS and to achieve the maintenance of fluid and electrolyte balance. In selected patients with rapid intestinal transit and dilated bowel, longitudinal intestinal lengthening and tailoring (LILT) and serial transverse enteroplasty (STEP) may provide some benefit. Clinical outcomes indicate similar results for both STEP and LILT procedures. In the absence of bowel dilation, segmental reversal of the small bowel may reduce parenteral nutrition (PN) requirements. Intestinal transplantation is the last option in cases where all previous surgical attempts have failed and where life-threatening complications of PN have occurred. The results of small bowel transplantation - once being disappointing because of the high rate of rejection - seem nowadays to be promising partially due to the improvements in immunosuppressive therapy (using alemtuzumab). Multivisceral transplantation, for multi-organ involvement (liver/small bowel) is performed in very few centers worldwide; more studies are needed to confirm the benefit of multivisceral transplantation for patients with SBS. Therapeutic manipulations towards the growth of tissue-engineered small intestine using stem cells and biopharmaceuticals are emerging therapeutic approaches, developed during the past decade; the effectiveness of these therapeutic strategies remains unproven.

Introduction

Short bowel syndrome (SBS) is a pathologic condition which is characterized by reduced intestinal length and diminished intestinal absorptive capacity mainly due to extensive surgical resection, congenital defect, or pathological process affecting the small bowel. Traditionally, it is believed to occur when more than half of the small intestine is resected. The most severe form of SBS is seen when approximately 30% or 100 cm of small bowel is left after an extensive enterectomy. During the last decade, a new term has been introduced in order to characterize the functional ability of the remaining small bowel. Intestinal failure (IF) rather depicts primarily the functional incapacity of the small bowel. In patients with IF, the length of the small bowel may be normal but its function is significantly altered, thereby reducing the absorption of nutrients. A small bowel with altered absorptive capacity of 120 cm long may function worse than a small bowel of 80 cm length which is better functioning. The exact prevalence of the SBS remains unknown, although an indirect estimation based on the number of the patients receiving total parenteral nutrition (TPN) at home retrieves a number of approximately 1 per million [1].

ETIOLOGY

The underlying cause leading to SBS varies among different age groups. For example in children, necrotizing enterocolitis, atresia, gastroschisis and midgut volvulus can produce IF. On the other hand, postoperative complications, trauma, Crohn's disease and mesenteric vascular disease produce IF in adults. The etiology of IF is briefly presented in Table 1 [2, 3].

Table 1. Etiology of intestinal failure in children and adults

Children	Adults
Atresia	Post-operative complications
Abdominal wall defects	Crohn's disease
Post traumatic resection	Radiation enteritis
Congenital SBS	Trauma
Cancer	Cancer
Necrotizing enterocolitis	Motility disorders
Midgut volvulus	Volvulus
Intussusception	Mesenteric vascular disease
Arterial/Venous thrombosis	
Venous Thrombosis	
Gastroschisis	
Crohn's disease	
Hirschsprung's disease	

SYMPTOMS AND PATHOPHYSIOLOGIC RESPONSE

Patients suffering from SBS due to any of the above etiologies, exhibit malnutrition and are prone to electrolyte disturbances. Moreover, alterations in the hormonal driven gastrointestinal motility and in bowel transition lead in intestinal functional impairment which is much dependent on the length and the absorptive capacity of the remaining intestine. Presence or absence of the colon is also an important factor in the course of the disease. The absorptive capacity the colon is approximately 5 to 6 liters per day. Avid absorption of water, sodium and chloride takes place here. The gastrocolic reflex plays a key role in slowing intestinal transition so that carbohydrates that have not been absorbed in jejunum can now be fermented by the colonic flora into short chain fatty acids. This procedure can salvage up to 500 kcals per day [4]. Unfortunately this is not the case for patients with an ileostomy, thus no colon in continuity, who exhibit a loss of large amount of gastrointestinal secretions.

Preservation of the ileocaecal valve is of paramount importance and this is particularly evident in patients where the valve has been surgically resected; small intestine dilation and bacterial overgrowth may lead in gastrointestinal bleeding, inflammation and D lactic acidosis [5]. The vast majority of the gastrointestinal secretions is absorbed in the terminal ileum. Fats, vitamin B_{12} and bile acids follow then the portal circulation towards the liver. Surgical resection of the ileum leads in malabsorption which is more evident if less than 1 meter of small bowel is left in situ.

Various compensatory mechanisms take place in the remaining part of the small intestine following extensive enterectomy. During this adaptation phase, epithelial hyperplasia along with a slight increase in the diameter of the ileum, are both part of the intestinal response to an extensive resection. Numerous hormonal mechanisms are also implicated in the mechanism of restoration of the absorptive capacity of the remaining part of the ileum. The adaptation phase may last up to 24 months after surgical resection [6].

Table 2. Signs and symptoms in SBS

Bloating
Cramping
Fatigue
Loss of bone mass
Visual disturbances
Foul-smelling stool
Heartburn
Pale greasy stools (steatorrhea)
Vomiting
Muscle spasms
Weakness
Loss of coordination
Swelling of lower extremities (edema)
Lactose intolerance

The main symptom of short bowel syndrome is diarrhea, leading to dehydration, malnutrition, and weight loss. Severe loss of fluid and electrolytes (sodium, potassium, and chloride), as well as loss of vitamins, minerals, and nutrients, produce life threatening problems if left untreated. Although the severity of symptoms may vary from person to person, these may include fatigue, steatorrhea, bloating, vomiting and depending on which vitamin or mineral is deficient, further symptom examples may include visual disturbances, muscle spasms, loss of coordination and loss of bone mass. Clinical symptoms are briefly presented on Table 2.

Surgical Management

The aim of surgery in patients with SBS is to restore the function of the small bowel and increase the available surface of the intestinal epithelium, thus improving the nutritional status of these patients. A multidisciplinary approach is required to carefully select patients for surgical treatment.

In an attempt to slow intestinal transit, a variety of surgical methods have been proposed, including the construction of intestinal valves, colon interposition and reversal of a segment of small bowel. The creation of intussuscepted valves has failed to provide any benefit in these patients as the majority of them required reoperation and removal of the valve due to severe obstructive symptoms [7]. Isoperistaltic colon interposition (first described in 1971) also failed to provide any benefit in patients with SBS [8]. In contrast, segmental reversal of the small bowel seems promising in the absence of bowel dilation. In a recent study by Beyer-Berjot et al. the creation of an antiperistaltic segment of approximately 10 cm long of small bowel achieved weaning of PN in approximately half of the patients (17 of 38 total) [9].

Small bowel dysmotility and bowel dilation often lead in bacterial overgrowth refractory to medical treatment. Surgical interventions such as simple tapering enteroplasty, Longtitudinal Intestinal Lengthening and Tailoring (LILT) and Serial Transverse Enteroplasty (STEP) have been used to increase the surface of the intestinal epithelium and to improve bowel dilation. Simple tapering enteroplasty is the surgical removal of a portion of the anti-mesenteric segment of the small bowel, usually using a stapling device. Blood supply to the remaining tabularized antimesenteric border is preserved. This procedure can be performed in patients with adequate small bowel length and bowel dilation [10].

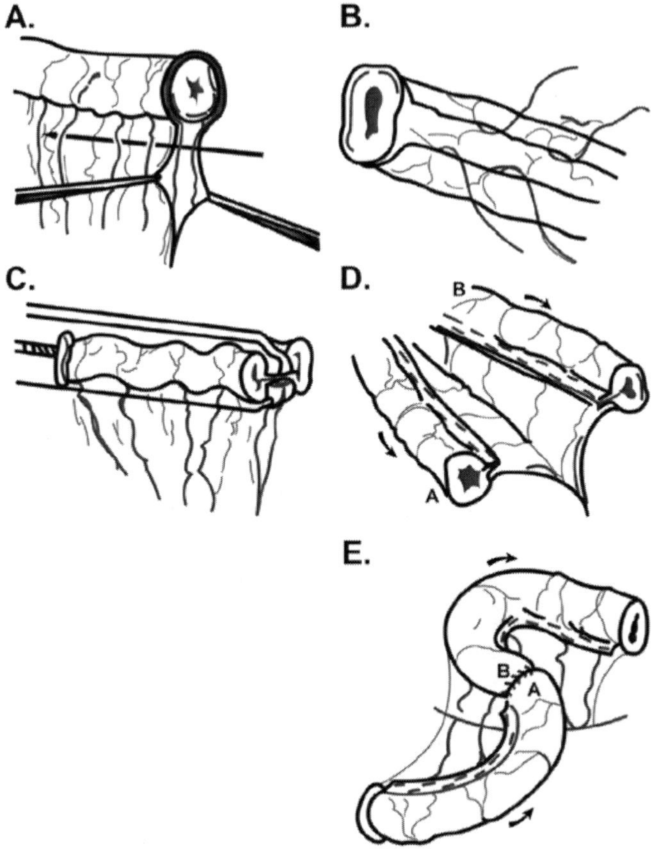

Figure 1. Steps in the LILT procedure as first described by Bianchi in 1980. A. Division of the mesentery B. Plane of the avascular space C. Division of the small bowel loop D – E the newly formatted bowel loops are anastomosed in a isoperistaltic fashion (with permission from reference 11).

In the LILT procedure the small bowel is divided longitudinally with care to preserve its arterial blood supply. The newly-created loops are anastomosed in an isoperistaltic fashion as shown in Figure 1 [11]. Limited data are available in adult patients regarding the results of the LILT procedure, although studies in pediatric patients have shown a clear benefit. Khalil et al. have shown that the overall survival rate was 92% in 19 patients following LILT procedure and the weaning from PN was reported to be over 90% [12]. A 10% rate of anastomotic stenosis has been reported by Devine et al. in patients who underwent LILT procedure [13].

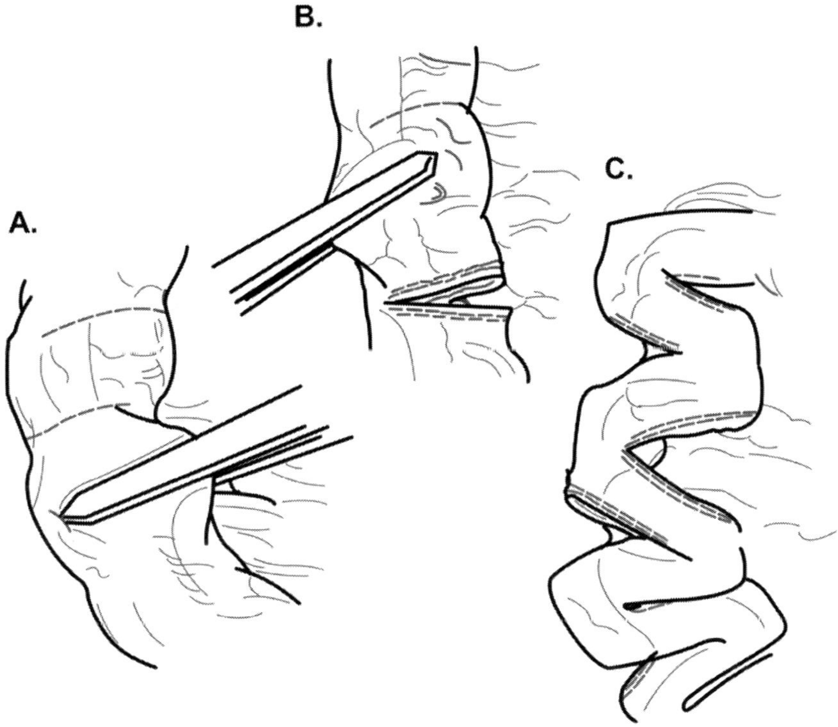

Figure 2. STEP procedure first described by Kim et al. in 2003. A-B A series of two staples are placed avoiding any arterial insult C. A zig zag formation of the lumen is established (with permission from reference 14).

Another promising surgical procedure is the serial transverse enteroplasty (STEP) first described in 2003 [14]. The luminal channel is given a zig zag format by firing transversally a series of staples with care to preserve intestinal blood supply, as shown in Figure 2. A recent 5-year study including 12 pediatric patients showed remarkably improved outcomes. About 65% of the patients avoided transplantation and seven patients achieved weaning from PN [15]. Another important study which included 29 patients with SBS who had undergone the STEP procedure showed a remarkable increase in the amount of intestinal caloric uptake [16].

Sudan et al. conducted a study (n = 64 patients, adults = 14) comparing the results of the STEP and LILT procedures [17]. Both procedures achieved similar results regarding avoidance of PN complications, with an overall survival rate of 91%. Stastistical analysis of these results failed to document the superiority of one technique over the other.

INTESTINAL TRANSPLANTATION

When all the above procedures have failed to treat SBS and to control life-threatening complications of PN, intestinal transplantation remains a salvage option. In 2000, the US Centers for Medicare and Medicaid Services (CMS) have approved intestinal transplantation as a treatment option for patients with SBS and PN failure [18]. Criteria for PN failure include:

1. Liver failure or PN liver disease
2. Thrombosis of central veins used for PN administration
3. ARDS, fungemia or sepsis related to PN administration
4. Recurrent dehydration and loss of metabolic homeostasis.

Absolute contraindications to small bowel transplantation include neurological disabilities and non-resectable malignancy. Multisystem autoimmune diseases and severe immunological deficiencies may be considered as relative contraindications.

Since intestinal transplantation is reserved for patients suffering life-threatening complications, prevention of rejection is of paramount importance.

Intestinal transplantation can be performed alone, in combination with liver transplantation, or as a part of a multivisceral transplantation. The prognosis is far better when the procedure is performed in the absence of liver failure [20]. One year survival rate and graft viability rate where reported to be as high as 89% and 72%, respectively [20]. Five-year graft survival rate has been reported to drop to 31% in children less than 1 year of age and to 69% in pediatric patients group aged from 6 to 10 years [21, 22, 23]. Leading causes of postoperative mortality are sepsis after rejection, respiratory failure, and multi-organ failure [20]. Acute rejection of the transplant should be differentiated from CMV infection or post-transplant lymphoproliferative disorder (PTLD) [24]. Preoperative comorbidity correlates inversely with transplant survival rates [25]. A promising scoring system has been proposed for preoperative risk assessment; however, this system should be validated in upcoming studies [26]. Alemtuzumab (anti CD52 monoclonal antibody) has shown sobering results that have spawned efforts towards immunosuppression [27]. Similar clinical outcomes have been reported when comparing the PN dependent patients group and intestinal transplantation patients group [28]. In addition, a recent study by Sudan et al. shows a better outcome in terms of quality living, in non-transplanted patients [29].

Emerging new therapies in the field of tissue engineering, aiming to achieve small intestine regeneration, may offer in the future an alternative therapeutic option to intestinal transplantation, thereby eliminating post-transplant morbidity [30, 31, 32, 33].

References

[1] Bakker H, et al. Home parenteral nutrition in adults: a european multicentre survey in 1997. ESPEN-Home Artificial Nutrition Working Group. *Clin Nutr* 1999;18:135e40.

[2] Thompson JS, DiBaise JK, Iyer KR, Yeats M, Sudan DL. Postoperative short bowel syndrome. *J Am Coll Surg* 2005; 201: 85-89.

[3] Goulet O, Ruemmele F. Causes and management of intestinal failure in children. *Gastroenterology* 2006; 130: S16-S28.

[4] DiBaise JK, Young RJ, Vanderhoof JA. Intestinal rehabilitation and the short bowel syndrome: part 2. *Am J Gastroenterol* 2004; 99:1823e32.

[5] Kaufman SS, et al. Influence of bacterial overgrowth and intestinal inflammation on duration of parenteral nutrition in children with short bowel syndrome. *J Pediatr* 1997;131:356e61.

[6] Dowling RH, Booth CC. Structural and functional changes following small intestinal resection in the rat. *Clin Sci* 1967;32:139e49.

[7] Waddell WR, et al. A simple jejunocolic "valve." For relief of rapid transit and the short bowel syndrome. *Arch Surg* 1970; 100:438e44.

[8] Glick PL, de Lorimier AA, Adzick NS, Harrison MR. Colon interposition: an adjuvant operation for short-gut syndrome. *J Pediatr Surg*. 1984;19:719-725.

[9] Beyer-Berjot L, Joly F, Maggiori L, et al. Segmental reversal of the small bowel can end permanent parenteral nutrition dependency: an experience of 38 adults with short bowel syndrome. *Ann Surg*. 2012;256:739-745.

[10] Weber TR, Vane DW, Grosfeld JL. Tapering enteroplasty in infants with bowel atresia and short gut. *Arch Surg*. 1982;117:684-688.

[11] Bianchi A. Intestinal loop lengthening—a technique for increasing small intestinal length. *J Pediatr Surg*. 1980;15:145-151.

[12] Khalil BA, Ba'ath ME, Aziz A, et al. Intestinal rehabilitation and bowel reconstructive surgery: improved outcomes in children with short bowel syndrome. *J Pediatr Gastroenterol Nutr*. 2012;54:505-509.

[13] Devine RM, Kelly KA. Surgical therapy of the short bowel syndrome. *Gastroenterol Clin North Am* 1989;18:603e18.

[14] Kim HB, Fauza D, Garza J, Oh JT, Nurko S, Jaksic T. Serial transverse enteroplasty (STEP): a novel bowel lengthening procedure. *J Pediatr Surg.* 2003;38:425-429.

[15] Oliveira C, de Silva N, Wales PW. Five-year outcomes after serial transverse enteroplasty in children with short bowel syndrome. *J Pediatr Surg.* 2012;47:931-937.

[16] Modi BP, et al. First report of the international serial transverse enteroplasty data registry: indications, efficacy, and complications. *J Am Coll Surg* 2007;204:365e71.

[17] Sudan D, et al. Comparison of intestinal lengthening procedures for patients with short bowel syndrome. *Ann Surg* 2007;246:593 – 604.

[18] https://www.cms.gov/medicare-coverage-database/details/ncd-details.aspx?NCDId=280&ncdver=2&DocID=260.5&SearchType=Advanced&bc = IAAAABAAAAAA& (accessed 11/5/2015).

[19] DeLegge M, et al. Short bowel syndrome: parenteral nutrition versus intestinal transplantation. Where are we today? *Dig Dis Sci* 2007;52: 876e92.

[20] Nishida S, Levi D, et al., Ninety-five cases of intestinal transplantation at the University of Miami, *J Gastrointest Surg*. 2002 Mar-Apr;6:233-9.

[21] Mazariegos GV, Steffick DE, Horslen S, et al. Intestinal transplantation in the United States 1999-2008. *Am J Transplant* 2010;10:1020–34.

[22] Grant D, Abu-Elmagd K, Reyes J, et al. 2003 report of the intestine transplant registry: a new era has dawned. *Ann Surg* 2005;241:607–13.

[23] Abu-Elmagd K, Costa G, Bond GJ, et al. Five hundred intestinal and multivisceral transplantations at a single center. *Ann Surg* 2009; 250:567–81.

[24] Wu T, Abu-Elmagd K, Bond G, Nalesnik MA, Randhawa P, Demetris AJ. A schema for histologic grading of small intestine allograft acute rejection. *Transplantation* 2003; 75: 1241-1248.

[25] Sivaprakasam R, Hidenori T, et al., Preoperative Comorbidity Correlates Inversely with Survival after Intestinal and Multivisceral Transplantation in Adults. *J Transplant*. 2013; Article ID 202410, 5 pages, doi:10.1155/2013/202410.

[26] Middleton SJ, Nishida S, et al. Cambridge-Miami score for intestinal transplantation preoperative risk assessment: initial development and validation, *Transplant Proc*. 2010;42:19-21.

[27] Nishida S, Levi DM, et al. Intestinal transplantation with alemtuzumab (Campath-1H) induction for adult patients, *Transplant Proc.* 2006;38:1747-9.
[28] Sudan DL. Treatment of intestinal failure: intestinal transplantation. *Nat Clin Pract Gastroenterol Hepatol.* 2007;4:503-510.
[29] Sudan D. Long term outcomes and quality of life after intestinal transplantation. *Curr Opin Organ Transplant* 2010;15:357–60.
[30] Grant CN, Mojica SG, et al. Human and mouse tissue-engineered small intestine both demonstrate digestive and absorptive function, *Am J Physiol Gastrointest Liver Physiol.* 2015;308:G664-77.
[31] Shaker A, Rubin DC, Intestinal stem cells and epithelial-mesenchymal interactions in the crypt and stem cell niche, *Transl Res.* 2010;156:180-7.
[32] Belchior GG, Sogayar MC, Grikscheit TC, Stem cells and biopharmaceuticals: vital roles in the growth of tissue-engineered small intestine, *Semin Pediatr Surg.* 2014 Jun;23:141-9.
[33] Spurrier RG, Grikscheit TC, Tissue engineering the small intestine, *Clin Gastroenterol Hepatol.* 2013;11:354 8.

Biographical Sketches

Dimitrios K. Nasikas, MD, MBS

Affiliation: PGY-4 Resident, Department of Surgical Oncology, Saint Savvas Cancer Hospital, Athens, Greece.

Date of Birth: 07/29/1982

Education: Medical degree, University of Crete (2010).
Master in Biomedical Sciences "Molecular Basis of Human Disease", University of Crete (2013).

Address: 6 Pythagora St, Paiania, Attica, Greece

Research and Professional Experience: PhD candidate, University of Crete (exp. 2018)

Honors: State Scholarships Foundation for academic excellence during year 5 and 6 of medical school (GPA: 10/10)

Publications Last 3 Years

[1] Dimitrios K Nasikas, Michael Sofopoulos, Niki Arnogiannaki, George H Sakorafas, C-cell hyperplasia as an incidental finding in a patient with papillary thyroid microcarcinoma, Int. J. Endo. Oncol. (2015) 2(4), 257–262.

[2] George H. Sakorafas, Dimitrios Nasikas, Dimitrios Thanos, Sotirios Gantzoulas, Incidental Thyroid C Cell Hyperplasia: Clinical Significance and Implications in Practice, Oncol Res Treat 2015;38:249–252.

[3] George H Sakorafas, Myrsini Gkeli, Victoria Kartsouni, Dimitra Daskalopoulou, Dimitrios Thanos, Dimitrios Nasikas, Sotirios Gantzoulas, Preoperatively diagnosed microscopic papillary thyroid cancer: an aggressive approach in selected patients with small nodules, Int. J. Endo. Oncol. (2015) 2(3), 241–247.

[4] George H Sakorafas, Konstantina K Katseni, Dimitrios Thanos, Dimitrios Nasikas, George Goutis, Parthenopi Deskoulidi, Thyroid cancer in a patient with congenital thyroid hemiagenesis, Int. J. Endo. Oncol. (2015) 2(2), 109–110.

George H. Sakorafas, MD, PhD

Affiliation: Chairman, Department of Surgical Oncology, Saint Savvas Cancer Hospital, Athens, Greece

Date of Birth: Sept 26, 1961

Education: Medical degree, Aristotle University of Thessaloniki (1985) Ph.D. Thesis: Oncogenes in the Cancer of the Pancreas (Athens University, Medical School, 1994)

Address: Arkadias 19-21, 115 26 Athens Greece
Tel/Fax + 30 210 7487192
Email:georgesakorafas@yahoo.com

Research and Professional Experience:

Assistant Professor of Surgery

Athens University, Medical School

Chairman, Department of Surgical Oncology, SAINT SAVVAS Cancer Hospital

Publications Last 3 Years

Dimitrios K Nasikas, Michael Sofopoulos, Niki Arnogiannaki, George H Sakorafas, C-cell hyperplasia as an incidental finding in a patient with papillary thyroid microcarcinoma, Int. J. Endo. Oncol. (2015) 2(4), 257–262.

George H. Sakorafas, Dimitrios Nasikas, Dimitrios Thanos, Sotirios Gantzoulas, Incidental Thyroid C Cell Hyperplasia: Clinical Significance and Implications in Practice, Oncol Res Treat 2015;38:249–252.

George H Sakorafas, Myrsini Gkeli, Victoria Kartsouni, Dimitra Daskalopoulou, Dimitrios Thanos, Dimitrios Nasikas, Sotirios Gantzoulas, Preoperatively diagnosed microscopic papillary thyroid cancer: an aggressive approach in selected patients with small nodules, Int. J. End. Oncol. (2015) 2(3), 241–247.

George H Sakorafas, Konstantina K Katseni, Dimitrios Thanos, Dimitrios Nasikas, George Goutis, Parthenopi Deskoulidi, Thyroid cancer in a patient with congenital thyroid hemiagenesis, Int. J. Endo. Oncol. (2015) 2(2), 109–110.

In: Short Bowel Syndrome (SBS)
Editor: Violet Chapman
ISBN: 978-1-63484-944-9

Chapter 2

SHORT BOWEL SYNDROME: CLINICAL FEATURES AND MANAGEMENT

José Antonio Rodríguez-Montes*, MD, PhD, FICS, Pedro J. Tárraga López, MD, PhD, and Juan Solera Albero, MD, PhD

ABSTRACT

Short bowel syndrome (SBS) refers to the malabsorptive state caused by physical and functional loss of portions of the small intestine, most frequently following extensive intestinal resection. Following resection, intestinal tissue undergoes morphological and functional changes to compensate for the losts function of the resected bowel, and extent of adaptation depends on resected bowel anatomy and the amount of remaining bowel. The clinical symptoms associated with SBS vary according to the length and location of the affected small bowel, the presence and nature of the underlying disease, and the presence or absence of the large bowel and ileocecal valve. The goals of medical treatment are to maintain fluid, electrolyte, and nutrient balances, as well as appropriate disease management to advoid side effects. In the past, all patients were managed on total parenteral nutrition at home. The development of medical therapies, such as recombinant growth hormone,

* Corresponding author: Prof. J.A. Rodríguez-Montes, Servicio de Cirugía General y del Aparato Digestivo, Hospital Universitario "La Paz", 5ª planta, Paseo de la Castellana, 261, 28046 Madrid. Spain, Email: rodriguezmontes@gmail.com.

octreotide and glucagon-like-peptide-2 analogs, has helped increases the intestinal absorption capacity. There are several surgical options to manage SBS. Technique choice depends on the patient´s underlying pathophysiology, and includes factors like intestinal transit time, remnant bowel length, presence of an intact colon, and degree of small bowel dilatation. Intestinal transplantation has been increasingly used with improving success in patients with intestinal failure life-threatening complications. We should continue to emphasize prevention of intestinal resection and conservation of as much intestine as possible in massive resection.

INTRODUCTION

Short bowel syndrome (SBS) is a common clinical problem for gastroenterologists, surgeons and other specialists who treat nutritional and gastrointestinal problems in children and adults. SBS-associated intestinal failure is a highly disabling condition that impairs quality of life and social integration. Despìte not being uniformly fatal, it may lead to serious life-threatening complications. The medical literature porposes various definitions for SBS and intestinal failure, but many focus on different aspects of these conditions, which is confusing. Thus, new definitions arise [1]: "intestinal failure results from obstruction, dysmotility, surgical resection, congenital defect, or disease-associated loss of absorption, and is characterized by the inability to maintain protein-energy, fluid, electrolyte, or micronutrients balance"; "short bowel syndrome results from surgical resection, congenital defect, or disease-associated loss of absorption, and is characterized by the inability to maintain protein-energy, fluid, electrolyte or micronutrient balances when on a conventionally accepted normal diet."

SBS occurs in patients who have had at least half of their small intestine removed, and somethimes all or part of their large intestine; or present a severely damaged intestine, dysmotility, or poor movement, inside intestines. SBS may be mild, moderate, or severe, depending on how well the small intestine works. SBS occurs in adults who have less than 200 cm of jejunum-ileum remaining after intestinal resection [2]. SBS patients cannot absorb enough water, vitamins, minerals, proteins, fat, calories, and other nutrients from food. What nutrients the small intestine has trouble in absorbing depend on what small intestine section has been damaged or removed.

ETIOLOGY AND EPIDEMIOLOGY

There are many causes of SBS [3, 4], the main form of surgery is to remove a portion of the small intestine. This surgery can treat intestinal diseases, injuries, or birth defects. Currently, mesenteric vascular accidents are the main cause in adults, followed by inflammatory bowel disease (Crohn´s disease), and radiation enteritis. In children, the main causes are congenital and perinatal diseases. Some children are born with an abnormally short small intestine or with part of their bowel missing, which can cause SBS. In infancy, SBS most commonly occurs following surgery to treat necrotizing enterocolitis, a condition in which part of the intestinal tissue is destroyed [5]. SBS may also occur following surgery to treat several pathologies: cancer and damage to the intestines caused by cancer treatment; inadverted gastroileostomy after gastric surgery; intestinal hernia; intestinal atresia; intestinal injury from trauma or from loss of blood flow due to a blocked blood vessel; intussusception; meconius ileus; midgut volvulus; omphalocele; intestinal neumatosis; gastroschisis, among others. Even if a person does not undergo surgery, disease or injury can damage the small intestine. Conditions that most frequently require the resection of a considerable length of small bowel are shown in Table 1. SBS incidence and prevalence are unknown because no reliable databases are available. Estimates are based on information from home parenteral nutrition (PN) registries, for which SBS is generally the most frequent indication. Two studies, limited to SBS patients, have reported the majority of patients being female and >50 years of age [6, 7]. A multifactorial etiology, uncertainly, intestinal length and varying definitions of SBS all make the comparing ofreports difficult. In the U.S., annual prevalence of home PN has been estimated to be aproximately 120 per million, of whom about 25% have SBS [8]. Each year SBS affects about three in every million people [5]. These numbers do not reflect patients with SBS who do not survive, were able to be weaned from PN during index hospitalization, or were able to be successfully weaned from home PN. Thus they, likely underestimate SBS prevalence.

SBS occurs in about 15% of adults who undergo intestinal resection; nearly 75% result from a single massive resection, and 25% from multiple resections [9]. Approximately 70% of those with newly acquired SBS are eventually able to be discharged from the hospital [10]. Reports have demonstrated 2-year and 5-year survival rates for SBS at over 80% and 70%, respectively [11, 12]. Survival rates are lower in the end-jejunal and ultrashort (remnant bowel 10% which an ileocecal valve, or 20% with no ileocecal valve) SB groups. PN dependence at 1, 2 and 5 years has been reported to be 74%, 64% and 48%, respectively [7]. In multivariate analyses, PN dependency lowered, with a remaining colon >57% and an SB remnant length >75 cm. In this study, over 25% of the patients who were eventually weaned completely from PN did so 2 years after their last bowel resection. Other factors which affect survival in SBS include patient's age, primary disease process, comorbid diseases, presence of chronic intestinal obstruction, and the experience of the team that manages the patient [13].

Table 1. Most frequent etiologies of short bowel syndrome

A) Organic pathologies which may require massive bowel resection
Adults
- Acute mesenteric ischaemia
- Intestinal volvulus
- Inflammatory bowel disease
- Diffuse neoplastic processes
- Diffuse poliposis
- Intestinal neoplasia
- Mesenteric injuries
- Radiactive enteritis
- Strangulated hernia (internal or external)
- Jejunocolic bypass or jejunoileal antiobesity (now in disuse)
- Adherence syndrome
- Gastroileostomy (unnoticed surgical error)
Children and newborns
- Intestinal atresia
- Intestinal volvulus
- Aganglionosis
- Gastroschisis
- Necrotizing enteritis
B) Situations that can behave as massive functional enterectomy
- High intestinal fistulas
- Derivations and high ostomy
- Chronic intestinal pseudoobstruction syndrome

PHYSIOPATOLOGY

Normal small bowel length in humans is 300-850 cm, and varies depending on the method used to measure it: X-ray, surgery or autopsy [13-15]. The duodenum occupies the first 25-30 cm, the jejunum some 160-200 cm, and the rest is the ileum [16]. When a resection of over 70-75% is done, or the length of the remaining intestine is <200 cm, SBS is considered to exist [2, 15]. Despite experience suggesting that patients with less than 200 cm of small intestine will quite likely develop intestinal failure, absorption does not depend only on residual intestine length as other prognostic factors exist, such as the quality of the remaining intestine, and presence or absence of a colon. In adults with no functional colon, dependence on total parenteral nutrition (TPN) persisting throughout life is likely if their residual intestine is less than 100 cm; if patients have an intact functional colon, dependence on TPN is likely to persist throughout life if their residual small intestine measures less than 60 cm. In breast-fed infants with SBS with only 10 cm of residual small intestine, not depending on TPN is normally achieved. Nonetheless, residual length is not the only factor that predicts enteral autonomy.

SBS clinics also depends on the small bowel anatomical region affected by resection or functional alteration [8, 16]. Most carbohydrate and protein absorption take place in the duodenum and jejunum [16], while the ileum is where fats and liposoluble vitamins (along with biliary salts excreted by the liver to the duodenum) are absorbed. The jejunum contains higher villi, deeper crypts and greater enzymatic activity than the ileum. Under normal conditions, 90% of the digestion and absorption of macro and micronutrients takes place in the initial 100-150 cm of the jejunum. Vitamin B_{12}, along with the intrinsic factor secreted into the stomach, is absorbed in the terminal ileum. Most fluids and electrolytes are absorbed in the ileum (80%) and the colon, and this implies the daily absorption of 2-3 litres of water and 7-9 litres of gastrointestinal secretions [3]. When intestinal resection affects the duodenum and/or the jejunum, the ileum can adapt to undertake its absorption functions, which is why resection is normally better tolerated if it affects the ileum.

The absorption of most nutrients can temporarily lower, which is compensated by ileal adaptation. While jejunal adaptation is only functional, ileal adaptation is so in structure and function terms [18, 19]. Yet despite ileal adaptation, enzymatic digestion can be affected by the irreplaceable loss of enteral hormones produced in the jejunum (cholecystokinin, secretin, GIP, VIP). Biliary and pancreatic secretions lower through lack of cholecystokinin and secretin, but gastrin levels increase through lack of GIP and VIP, which leads to gastric acid hypersecretion. Acid leaving the stomach can damage intestinal mucosa, while a low intraluminal pH produces unfavorable conditions for the activity of the pancreatic enzymes present. If malabsorbed nutrients reach the ileum and colon, their high osmolar load can cause osmotic diarrhea. Ileal resection consequences relate with another characteristic of the jejunum and ileum: ileal mucosa has "adapted" intercellular bindings, which allows it to concentrate lumen contents; however, jejuna mucosa possesses "porous" intercellular bindings, and the osmolarity of lumen contents is similar to plasmatic contents [18]. This enables the jejunum to rapidly move water and electrolytes through its mucosa from plasma to the intestinal lumen to suitably dilute lumen contents. As a result, fluids are secreted in the jejunum as a response to any hypertonic food, which is re-absorbed in the ileum, and also in the colon, but to a lesser extent. Thus an ileal resection of >100 cm causes loss of fluids and electrolytes. Other aspects that determine the severity of malabsorption are: 1) presence or absence of an intact colon as it is well able to absorb large quantities of liquids and electrolytes, and performs a very important, yet minor, function, in assimilating nutrients as it absorbs short-chain fatty acids; 2) less malabsorption is believed to occur with an intact ileocecal valve as this valve delays the transit of chyme from the small intestine to the colon; so it prolongs the time of contact between nutrients and small intestine mucosa; 3) a healthy residual small intestine reduces the degree of malabsorption severity; 4) a jejunum resection is better tolerated than an ileum one because the capacity of the latter to absorb biliary salts and vitamin B_{12} is specific.

Malabsorption in SBS patients worsens with gastric acid hypersecretion associated with hypergastrinemia, which persists 1-2 years after surgery. An increase in acid in the duodenum inhibits absorption by various mechanisms, among others, digestive enzyme inhibition, most of which act under alkalinity conditions. Clinically speaking, the adaptation period presents smaller volumes of, but frequent, defecations, a better capacity to assimilate enteral nutrients and the need for TPN is lower. Knowing the mechanisms that intervene in intestinal adaptation sometimes allows strategies to enhance adaptation to be established in SBS patients who cannot be weaned from TPN. Intestinal adaptation mechanisms in human patients are still not fully known.

PROGNOSTIC FACTORS

The main factors involved in the prognosis of SBS-related bowel failure include the anastomotic region of the resected bowel, residual bowel length, presence of an underlying pathology, presence or absence of a colon and of the ileocecal valve, the nature of the main disease [3] and the patient's age [20].

Residual bowel length correlates with the patient's degree of nutritional autonomy; that is, independence of PN. Patients with a very short residual bowel length are more likely to develop kidney failure [21] and liver failure [22], and depend more easily on PN. Intestinal resections that affect less than 33% do not imply protein-calorie malnutrition; loss of up to 50% allow nutritional tolerance with no nutritional support; those over 75% probably require PN to avoid malnutrition [17].

The anatomy of the remnant bowel, that is, if a colon or ileum continues, also affects the prognosis. Patients who are at high risk of losing nutritional autonomy are those with duodenostomy, <35 cm of residual jejunum in patients with jejunal-ileal anastomosis, <60 cm of residual bowel in patients with jejuno-colic or ileal-colic anastomosis, or <115 cm remanent with terminal jejunostomy [23]. Survival has been negatively correlated with terminal enterostomies, bowel length <50 cm and with intestinal infarct as the cause, but not with dependence on PN [23].

Functionality does not depend only on length; 150 cm of pathological intestine can function worse than 75 cm of healthy intestine. Some definitions of SBS and intestinal failure have been based on measures of the remnant bowel's functional capacity. These measures include loss of fecal energy [24], [25], or citrulline plasma levels [26, 27]. Citrulline is a product of the metabolism by the enterocyte of glutamine and derived amino acids which, on an empty stomach, can be synthesized by only the small intestine, and cannot be incorporated into body proteins. So on an empty stomach, citrulline plasma levels should provide a good functional mass index of residual enterocytes.

Ileocecal valve loss is a major factor in patients who have undergone ileal resection. The ileocecal valve acts as the main barrier against colic reflux from the colon to the small intestine, and helps regulate not only the fluids and nutrients that leave the ileum to the colon. If the ileocecal valve is intact, intestinal transit slows down, but experimental studies have questioned this fact [28]. Resection of the terminal ileum and ileocecal valve is associated with bacterial overgrowth, a relevant aspect of SBS.

If the colon remains, it can sometimes prove to be a critical determining factor for patients who are independent of IV support because the colon in

SBS patients becomes a major digestion organ. The colon helps maintain fluids and electrolytes as it can increase its absorption capacity 5-fold after small intestine resection. It is also able to absorb proteins and retrieve malabsorbed carbohydrates through bacterial metabolism, which converts them into short-chain fatty acids [25]. The colon slows down intestinal transit and stimulates intestinal adaptation. Regarding PN dependence, presence of at least half a colon is the equivalent of 50 cm of small intestine [3]; thus patients can be grouped into two subgroups: those with a continuous colon (that is, jejunum-colon or jejunum-ileum-colon) and those with no colon, in whom a short bowel will end in stoma (enterostomy). With these beneficial effects, presence of a colon increases the incidence of calcium oxalate renal lithiasis. Oxalate is normally bound to calcium in the small intestine and becomes unsoluble when it reaches the colon; the colon is also necessary to produce SBS-related D-lactic acidosis, caused by malabsorbed carbohydrates being fermented into D-lactate in the colon, and this metabolite being absorbed and characterized by varying degrees of neurological symptoms [29].

Small Bowel Syndrome Types

There are three SBS patient groups depending on the type of anastomosis and whether the colon is present or not [3]. The first group is formed by those patients for whom resection affects part of the jejunum, ileum and colon, and they present terminal jejunostomy. The second group is formed by patients who have undergone ileal resection, which often involves the ileocecal valve, and thus have jejunal-colic anastomosis. Finally, other patients predominantly display jejunal resection with more than 10 cm of terminal ileum and remnant colon (jejunal-ileal). This last group of patients is quite scarce, whose management is similar to those with jejunal-colic anastomosis. Thus both groups enter the series of patients with SBS and preserved colon.

Patients with jejunostomy can, in turn, be grouped into "net absorbers " or "net secretors." "Net absorbers" absorb more water and sodium from their diet than what they orally take. They can be treated with oral water and sodium supplements, do not require parenteral fluids, and tend to have a remnant ileum of over 100 cm. Conversely, "net secretors" normally have a remnant ileum of less than 100 cm and lose more water and sodium through the stoma than they are capable of orally taking. Deficient jejunostomy in these patients considerably increases during the day in response to intake, and to a minimum at nighttime [14]; this secretory response can be reduced with gastric antisecretory drugs and octreotide, but can condition dependence on parenteral fluids.

INTESTINAL ADAPTATION

Following resection, intestinal tissue undergoes morphological and functional changes to compensate for lost resected bowel function (Table 2). These changes are mediated by multiple interactive factors, including intraluminal and parenteral nutrients, gastrointestinal regulatory peptides, hormones, cytokines and growth factors, many of which have been well characterized in animal models [30, 31], in addition to tissue factors that include immunity, blood flow and neural influences [32, 35]. Although the adaptative capacity of the ileum is greater than that of the jejunum, massive ileal resection has a significantly worse impact than jejunal resection as the ileum plays a key role in electrolyte and water absorption, and in the absorption of vitamin $B_{12,}$ bile salts and fatty acids. The amount of remaining small bowel is the most important predictor of the adaptative potential; neither structural nor functional adaptative changes have been demonstrated in human or animal models, and more extreme resections result in end-jejunostomy [35]. Bowel adaptation is a remodeling process which, involve compensatory mechanisms that aim to improve the remanent bowel´s absorptive capacity following intestinal loss. Increased intestinal mass and surface area occur through enterocyte and crypt cell proliferation, increase in microvilli with taller villi and deeper crypts, and hyperplasia and hypertrophy of smooth muscle layers [33 - 36]. Adaptation is an ongoing process that begins 24-48 h after surgical resection, and rapidly progresse during the initial 4-24 months following intestinal loss, and can even take years to complete [7, 37]. Following intestinal resection, the bowel´s motor activity is also disrupted for a few months [38]. Studies have demonstrated a shorter duration of the migratin motor complex cycle and feed pattern after resection [39]. Once this initial phase is over, motor adaptation results in a prolonged intestinal transit time and improved absorption by individuals enterocytes. In some patients, rapid bowel growth results in an excessively dilatated the remnant bowel which, in turn, results in dysmotility and stasis, both of which promote bacterial translocation with systemic infections, and liver injury [40, 41]. This may further negatively impact ongoing adaptation and, thus, the ability to wean PN [20]. Since bowel dilatation is a natural sequel of adaptation, surgery should be deferred unless dilatation causes recurrent episodes of bacteriemia

[42]. Bowel dilatation occurs more commonly in younger patients, who are more often candidates for surgical rehabilitation than adults [43].

Table 2. Intestinal structural and functional adaptative changes after massive small bowel resection

Structural
- Villus lengthening and expansion in microvilli
- Increased crypt cell depth and enterocyte number
- Increased gut muscle thickness, circumference and length
- Increased intestinal wet weight, protein and DNA
- Remnant bowel dilatation and elongation
Functional
- Up-or down-regulation of carrier-mediated transport
- Modified brush border membrane enzyme activity, fluidity and permeability
- Slowing of transit in the rat to allow prolonged time for absorption to occur
Others
- Fecal microbioma
- Bowel motor activity
- Immune functions?

The fecal microbiome in patients with SBS differs from that of healthy individuals. Stools from SBS patients accumulate significantly more bacterial classes *Gammaproteobacteria* and *Bacilli*. Differences in the composition and function of gut microbiomes in children with SBS may affect bowel physiology. These findings may provide new intestinal rehabilitation and clinical management opportunities [44].

For the adaptation process, presence of nutrients inside the intestinal lumen is important. So beginning with oral or enteral nutrition must start as soon as possible. Nutrients also provide substrates to reproduce enterocytes and can stimulate the release of trophic factors. It has been suggested that glutamine, short-chain fatty acids, unsaturated fats, ornithine and nucleotides can be an important luminal stimulus for such adaptation [45-48]. Glutamine is the basic energy substrate of enterocytes and a substrate for nucleic acids synthesis. However, the beneficial effects of their oral or IV supplementation during the adaptation process have not been clearly demonstrated [49, 50]. Polyamines (spermine, espermidine and putrescine) are regulators of intestinal adaptation and are synthesized in large quantities by rapidly proliferating tissues, as in the intestinal epithelium during adaptation. It has been experimentally demonstrated that enteral diets supplemented with alpha-ketoglutarate ornithine, a precursor of arginine, glutamine and polyamines, improve intestinal adaptation [51].

Intestinal adaptation can be stimulated by secretions and gastrointestinal hormones. Eating induces their release. Glucagon-like peptide-2 (GLP-2) is an enterotrophic, antisecretory and modulatory hormone of intestinal transit considered the main hormonal stimulus for intestinal adaptation, and is secreted by L-cells in the terminal ileum and colon in response to food intake. One of the mechanisms that could explain the beneficial effects of GLP-2 would be to activate the formation of decarboylase ornithine, a polyamine synthesis rate-limiting enzyme [52]. Resistant analogs to dipeptidyl peptidase, e.g., Teduglutide, have demonstrated improved absorption in these patients [53, 54]. Other hormones that can contribute to the adaptation process are enteroglucagon, epidermal growth factor, keratinocyte growth factor (KGF), growth hormone, cholecystokinin, gastrin, neurotensin, insulin, leptin and IGF-I [3, 30, 31, 48, 50, 51]. Hormones with antitrophic effects include: transforming growth factor beta-1 (TGF B-1), which inhibits precursor cells in intestinal mucosa in rats, wheras octreotide alters intestinal adaptation by reducing cellular proliferation [3]; ghrelin, whose levels tend to be low in SBS patients, the meaning of which remains unknown [55]. Prostaglandins also stimulate intestinal proliferation. Thus reducing their synthesis with acetyl-salicylic acid, non steroid anti-inflammatories or corticoids can inhibit the adaptation process.

Massive intestinal resections also determine changes in both the function and structure of gastric mucosa, and mucosa hyperchlorhydria and erosion stand out. Hyperchlorhydria agrees with the increase in oxyntic cells observed in gastric body glands. In dogs these oxyntic cells are bigger and more numerous, and they also present increased vesicles, which indicate greater activity, that occasionally constitute long tubular formations; conversely, mitochondria appear well conserved. The most interesing piece of evidence lies in the variations undergone in stomach endocrine cells, more specifically in G-cells or gastrin cells as EC, ECL, D, D1, L, SM and A apparently remain normal [56].

Intestinal adaptation can be facilitated because the patient eats more than is normal (hyperphagia), and the intestine is also able to adapt to accomplish more efficient absorption per surface unit by increasing its absorptive surface and/or slowing down gastrointestinal transit. Hyperphagia is a fundamental mechanism in humans, which occurs in more than 80% of SBS patients (>1,5 times basal energy usage levels). This negatively correlates with fat absorption and with BMI, and is not curbed by presence of parenteral nutrition. Over time, food intake in early stages increases and protein absorption improves.

Bacterial Overgrowth

Small intestine bacterial overgrowth (SIBO) appears when intestinal flora regulatory mechanisms alter, which helps colic-type flora proliferate in the small intestine which, in turn, alters absorption and digestion. The most frequently found species in SIBO cases are Streptococcos, Bacteroides, Escherichia and Lactobacillos. After intestinal resection, motility alters, which predisposes to bacterial overgrowth in the remnant bowel. The surgical removal of the ileocecal valve also allows colic-type bacteria to enter the small intestine; other factors that increase the risk of SIBO are using gastric antisecretory antidiarrheal drugs, presence of blind loop syndrome (e.g., in Billroth II-type anastomosis) and underlying processes such as chronic pseudo-obstruction [3].

SIBO has a strong negative impact on digestion and nutrients absorption as bacteria compete with enterocytes for nutrients. Fat malabsorption takes place in SIBO, as do steatorrhea and lack of liposoluble vitamins A, D and E in clinical terms; no vitamin K shortage occurs because it is synthetized by intestinal bacteria. Vitamina B_{12} is also malabsorbed and megaloblastic anemia sets in when cobalamin binds to the bacteria in the proximal intestine; inactive vitamin B_{12} analogs increase in SIBO, and its catabolism increases to inactive cobamides through the action of some bacteria *(Clostridium, Escherichia coli* and *Propionibacterium).* Folic acid levels are normal or high as bacteria are capable of synthesizing this acid [3]. Carbohydrate absorption also alters, which is especially due to intraluminal consumption and to the reduction in local disaccharidases (lactase and sucrase) given the lesion caused by bacteria to mucosa; protein malabsorption may also occur through intraluminal catabolism and poor absorption. Besides altered absorption, SIBO can bring about inflammatory alterations in intestinal mucosa, which increases not only its permeability, but also the risk of bacterial translocation and sepsis. Inflammation can cause anastomotical ulcers, and acute or chronic intestinal hemorrhaging, which leads to microcytic anemia, and to other alterations like hepatic steatosis and exacerbated hepatotoxicity in connection with PN [57]; it has also been related with the risk of intestinal neoplasias through the production of carcinogenic substances, specifically with colon cancer, perhaps due to excess biliary acids. SIBO presents diverse clinical effects whose severity varies.

The objective of treating SIBO is to modify bacterial flora by cutting the number of pathogenic bacteria without forgetting that normal bacterial flora must remain. As no controlled assays exist for SIBO treatment in SBS patients, recommendations are made based on clinical experience. Antibiotic treatment is empirical and covers anaerobic and aerobic bacteria. A 10-14-day cycle with oral antibiotics (e.g., metronidazole or tetracicline) should improve symptoms (meteorism, diarrhea, weight loss) in 1-2 weeks [3]; some patients, e.g., those with chronic pseudo-obstruction, require constant treatment. So it is advisable to rotate antibiotics in order to avoid the overgrowth of resistant bacteria, and to determine antibiotic sensitivity if they do not respond positively to antibiotic therapy. Apart from using antibiotics, reconsidering the prescription of antisecretory and antimotility drugs might be a useful measure as the elimination of these drugs can be beneficial in some patients. Using prebiotics has also been recommended [58].

Nutritional support is a relevant aspect in SIBO treatment, especially when we consider that its presence may require PN. Restricting carbohydrates to reduce associated gases and osmotic diarrhea, and increasing protein and fat intake, are advisable [3]. It is necessary to bear in mind that high fat intake in patients who have lost biliary salts can make diarrhea worse, and can also increase the risk of oxalate-related lithiasis. Other options to control SIBO, which include intermittent gastric lavage with ethylene glycol or prescribing anti-inflammatories in patients with serious inflammation, are not conclusive and are not, thus, routinely used.

CLINICAL MANIFESTATIONS

The clinical symptoms of a patient with a short bowel generally come in three phases, and are summarized in Table 3 [59].

Since virtually all the components that are useful for the organism, and most of water and electrolytes, are absorbed by the small intestine, the potential spectrum of short bowel clinical symptoms is almost infinite [60], [61]. The absorption of almost all nutrients is poor and, with time, this circumstance implies serious weight loss, tiredness, laxness and weakness as a result of the disorders that derive from poor fat, glycide and protein absorption.

Table 3. Clinical course of SBS

PHASE 1.- Initial period
Characterized by:
- Loss of liquids and electrolytes (vomiting and diarrhea)
- 5-10 bowel movements/day (dehydratation, hypovolemia and acidosis)
- Anorectal abrasions
- Weight loss (13-30%)
PHASE 2.- Progressive adaptation
Characterized by:
- Less diarrhea
- Appetite comes back
- Intestinal function become normal
- Compensatory mechanisms appear
PHASE 3.- Equilibrium period (6-24 months post-resection)
Characterized by:
- Fewer bowel movements (2-4/day)
- Stable weight (70-90% of initial weight)
- Frequent anemia (hypochromic, megaloblastic, mixed)
- Temporarily diminished libido
- Normal puberty
- Symptoms of tetany
- Osteoporosis and osteomalacia
- Neuropsychiatric alterations
- Skin-mucosa lesions

Hypochromic and megaloblastic anemias, or mixed anemias, are not rare when prophylactic iron and vitamin B_{12} are lacking.

In adults, secondary sexual characters persist after resection, but tend to temporarily diminish libido.

Symptoms of tetany are frequent, mainly due to hypocalcemia. However, hypomagnesemia can favour or prolong them, although it is masked by normal serum magnesium. Presence of hypophosphatasemia is also known.

Osteoporosis, osteopenia and osteomalacia result from uncorrected chronic hypocalcemia, and are associated with long-term protein malnutrition, and possibly with hypovitaminosis. Yet other factors can influence, such as medication, gender, ethnic race, body size and little sun exposure [62].

Group B vitamins, and isolated cases of vitamin B_{12} and vitamins A and C, have been described as lacking. Purpura and generalized hemorrhaging may reflect alterations in coagulation caused by vitamin K malabsorption. Presence of hypoproteinemia has also been reported.

Neuropsychiatric alterations can vary: sleepiness, psychosis, hyporeflexia, paresthesias, etc [63]. Skin-mucosa alterations secondary to hypovitaminosis A and B are not unusual: rhagades, glossitis, stomatitis, pellagra and alterations in skin appendages.

The seriousness of gastrointestinal sequelae from SBS depends on several factors: length and anatomical location of the residual bowel, presence or absence of the ileocecal value, concomitant colic disease, mucosa integrity, residual bowel function, and time since the syndrome appeared.

COMPLICATIONS WITH SBS

The most frequent complications with SBS are listed in Table 4. In later stages, we can come across anemia, deteriorated nutritional status, and lack of fatty acids, vitamins and minerals. Iron absorption becomes more difficult when the patient has lost duodenal and jejunal mucosa. Calorie-protein malnutrition and loss of macro/micronutrients and trace elements appear. Severe teething alterations may occur in pediatric patients.

Parenteral lipid and liposoluble vitamin requirements need to be independently determined because fat absorption may be suitable, which prevents loss of essential fatty acids, but poor absorption of liposoluble vitamins A, D, E and K may appear with major loss in ileal length, and also with limited fat absorption. Malabsorption of biliary acids and the subsequent depletion of the biliary acids pool increase the chances of gallstones forming. Selenium has been reported to be lacking in patients with a short bowel, which should be routinely administered.

Special attention should be paid to lactic acidosis and nephrolithiasis secondary to calcium oxalate calculi. Lactic acidosis can be life-threatening. Lactic acid is caused by bacterial overgrowth, which appears particularly when the ileocecal valve is missing. Humans lack the enzyme needed to metabolize D-lactic acid. To cut the risk of lactic acidosis, correcting dehydration is most important while administering sodium citrate supplements and restricting fat and oxalate in the patient's diet. The clinical supplementary use of *Oxalobacter formigenes* to enhance the destruction of oxalate or cholestyramine to ligate oxalate is still far from being conclusive [8].

Table 4. Most frequent SBS complications

- Anemia
- Bone disease
- Diarrhea (cholerrheic/steatorrheic)
- D-lactic acidosis
- Hypomagnesemia
- Calorie-protein malnutrition
- Lack of trace elements
- Lack of vitamins (A, D, E, K and B12)
- Depletion of biliary salts
- Cholelithiasis
- Dehydratation
- Hypocalcemia
- Hepatic fibrosis
- Renal lithiasis (oxalates)

D-lactic acid serum levels can be found at high levels, and can cause marked acidosis and behavioral changes. In these circumstances, providing a basis for nutritional support with no oral intake is necessary until oral antibiotics can prevent the source of acidosis from occurring. Managing carbohydrate intake as a treatment for lactic acidosis has been recommended rather than submitting pediatric patients to repeated antibiotic treatments.

Calcium oxalate calculi in kidneys come secondary to a rise in serum oxalate levels, which is usually linked to calcium in the intestinal lumen and is eliminated. Apparently, colic mucosa in SBS is exposed to higher oxalate levels because luminal calcium is linked to non absorbed biliary acids and is, therefore, not available to link the oxalate found in the lumen. It would seem that mucosa is more permeable to oxalate due to the detergent effect of biliary acids and free fatty acids.

Complications appear in patients who undergo prolonged TNP, including liver disease and cholelithiasis, and biliary sludge is the most frequent, which possibly has the clinical consequences of cholecystitis, choledocholithiasis and pancreatitis [8, 59]. As cholelithiasis appears to be more frequent in SBS patients than in the general population, prophylactic cholecystectomy has been recommended [64]. Both administration of more than 1 g/kg/day of parenteral lipids and presence of cholestasis have been associated with liver complications [22]. For patients who depend on PN, "intestinal rehabilitation" methods have been designed to enhance the remnant bowel's capacity to absorb.

Acute and chronic complications related with PN infusion catheters are well-known, like those that derive from: catheter insertion and care; PN formula; incorrect administration [43, 65].

In order to know the progress made in patients with a short bowel, a serum and urine analysis with 3-methyhistidine, polyamine, ATP hydrolysis and calcium kinetics, has been proposed. It has been concluded that the post-absorptive concentration of citrulline in plasma is a marker of the remnant bowel's absorption function, and that it is a good indicator of intestinal failure in SBS patients after a 2-year adaptation period [26, 27].

MEDICAL TREATMENT

The object of medically treating patients with a short bowel is to optimize their nutrient assimilation and to prevent complications with TPN and sequelae from chronic malabsorption. As previously mentioned, the evolution of SBS patients comes in three phases, whose treatment priorities in each one differ.

During the immediate post-operatory period, electrolytes and nutritional status have to be frequently monitored. This period tends to cover 7-10 days, and can last 1 month; the second phase is stabilization (which lasts 1-3 months) when intestinal adaptation develops to compensate for the reduced absorption surface. Finally, the third phase starts after 3 months and ends in intestinal adaptation.

Although some sequelae and forms of treatment are common to all three SBS phases, treatment should be taken on an individual basis by taking the basic pathology, morbidity, functional residual capacity, and even the patient's prognosis, into account [59, 61].

Initial post-operatory treatment must be based on correct fluids-electrolytes balance. Recommended replacement patterns vary, although the use of glucose and maltodextrins, along with sodium, in standard oral rehydration seem to improve sodium absorption. If lost electrolytes are not adequately replaced, hypovolemia, hypotension, and frequently intestinal ischemia, can take place in patients with marginal splanchnic perfusion. Among others, it is vital to monitor hemodynamic parameters, and even pulmonary pressures in some cases. Sodium must be monitored very carefully as sodium loss is great in this phase (8-100 mEq/L). Lack of zinc through gastrointestinal secretions might entail administering supranormal doses in SBS patients.

Pharmacologically treating diarrhea can start early to help reduce loss of fluids and electrolytes. Octeotride is employed as a gold standard drug to control hydroelectrolytic loss; this analog of somatostatin drastically reduces gastrointestinal and billiopancreatic secretions, although its main drawback is it produces biliary sludge, and even cholelithiasis. It also entails the risk of causing intestinal ischemia given its mesenteric flux depressor effect. Adult SBS patients who depend on PN and/or IV delivered fluid supports have two pharmacological treatment options which can favour intestinal growth: glucagon-like peptide 2 analog (teduglutide) and somatotropin, a recombinant human growth hormone. Teduglutide improves absorption [65], but has adverse gastrointestinal effects, such as abdominal distension, abdominal pain and nausea. Somatotropin reduces PN requirements and its most common place side effects are peripheral edemas and musculo-skeletal episodes [65].

All SBS patients must take gastric antisecretory drugs, such as H_2 receptor antagonist drugs or proton pump inhibitors, in order to neutralize hyperclorhydria induced by SBS [61]. Other agents used during the immediate post-operatory period include opiates and antimotility/cholestyramine drugs.

A priority in this SBS phase is to preserve the venous system as it is the main way to nutrition, hydratation and medication. Il use and abuse of surface veins can cause thrombosis and must always be avoided. The best way to conserve the venous system is to place a long-term catheter as soon as SBS has been established.

TPN should commence early to obtain a positive nitrogenated balance and to avoid serious weight loss, and must continue until adaptation processes have been completed, or should be indefinitely continued if clinical circumstances require it. Carefully estimating calorie requirements is perceptive and must be repeated frequently whenever the patient's condition requires it. Initially, monitoring must be done daily until the patient becomes stable, and then becomes less frequent, but will always be an important measure.

In the intermediate phase, adaptation must continue to compensate the reduced absorption surface, and alternating fat absorption, calcium, magnesium and vitamins must persist. The treatment priority in this phase includes ensuring nutrient and fluid requirements, and beginning enteral or oral nutrition. Glutamine will be provided parenterally and enterally.

In the chronic phase, oral diet will be the main form of nutrition. In certain cases, due to resection length or the residual bowel pathology, it is not feasible to reach a sufficient degree of adaptation and PN needs to continue.

These patients need a calorie intake of 35 kcal/kg/day. Protein needs are estimated to be 1-1,5 g protein/kg/day and glycide intake at 2,5-4 mg/kg/min, with a maximum of 5 g/kg/day. Fat intake must be 1-1,5 g/kg/day until 10-50% of the total [59].

SBS patients with an intact colon should eat diets rich in glycides, but poor in fat and oxalate; suitable monthly doses of vitamin B_{12} must be administered to patients with a resected ileum length over 100 cm, and PN must be used only when eating cannot be performed orally or enterally.

Nutritional intake according to resected bowel length is [59, 66]:

a) <30% (<100 cm). Nutritional consequences are minimum and patients may also require cholestyramine to absorb biliary acids and vitamin B_{12}.
b) 30-50% (100-200 cm). If the ileum has been removed, diet must be low-fat and cholestyramine will be prescribed.
c) >50% (>200 cm). Progressive enteral nutrition may be indicated and TPN must be administered.
d) >75% (>300 cm). TPN is preceptive. If the remnant small intestine is <80 cm long-term TPN is probably needed. Another option is surgical treatment. If there is a serious hepatic problem due to long-term TPN administration, a simultaneous liver and intestine (combined) transplantation is a possibility.

Surgical Treatment

Surgically treating SBS is a therapeutic option that must be put into practice only when first-choice medical-diet treatment is not able to achieve acceptable patient nutritional status, serious complications appear because of the patient's condition which entails having to suspend this treatment, or the patient's quality of life with this treatment becomes untolerable.

The following general considerations about surgically treating SBS can be made:

The surgeon must undertake SBS prophylaxis when faced with a situation that implies massive intestinal resection. Exereses must be limited as much as possible (especially when they affect the ileum), the ileocecal valve must also be respected if at all possible, and termino-terminal anastomosis is recommended to avoid blind loop syndrome as this can harm compensation mechanisms. If the patient on resection treatment is a carrier of previous digestion bypasses that can help establish SBS, the suitability of eliminating them during the same surgical treatment must be assessed.

None of the operations considered in this epigraph must be done during responsible SBS resection surgery as the intestinal adaptation potential can render them unnecessary. Yet many of the techniques assayed in experimental surgery conduct intestinal resection and the procedure is used to relieve potential SBS following exeresis during the same surgical procedure.

Nor should surgical treatment be practiced in the initial syndrome phase, but after at least 6-12 months following resection and when patients cannot maintain 70% of their normal weight without PN; that is, in the last disease stage to allow mechanisms of compensation to be fully completed in the remnant bowel [67].

An intestine transplantation is the ideal solution to treat SBS. Yet despite the advances made in its outcome, it is not routinely used in human clinics.

Numerous surgical procedures to relieve the consequences of extensive intestinal resection have been devised [68-90], but many have not been employed in human clinics and have remained in the experimental surgery field.

The surgical techniques available to treat SBS are offered in Table 5 where they are grouped according to their objective.

For SBS patients, surgery can play an important role in preventing, migrating and, in some cases, reversing intestinal failure. During intestinal resection, bowel length should be conserved to the fullest possible extent to advoid dependence of PN. Bowel salvage may be improved by initially preserving tissue of questionable viability and later reassessing by "second look" procedures. Once patients are stabilized, ostomy reversal and recruitment of distal unused bowel should be prioritized whenever feasible. Following progression to intestinal failure, surgical SBS management depends on the symptoms and anatomical characteristics of each individual patient.

The mainstay of management for children with SBS includes a prolonged course of PN and dietary adjustaments until a degree of intestinal adaptation that is compatible with life and sustained growth has been achieved [88]. These include vagotomy and piloroplasty, recirculating small bowel loops, reversed small bowel segments (single and paired), periintestinal rings, pouch formation, and prejejunal or preileal colon transposition. Other researchers have attempted to grow small intestinal mucosa on colonic serosal patches, or have used vascularized abdominal wall pedicle flaps, mucosal denuded tubular colonic segments and prosthethic materials, bowel elongation techniques, neomucosa growth, among others. Experimental models for small bowel transplantation have also been developed, although clinical application is presently not routine.

Table 5. Procedures resorted to for treating SBS

Techniques to increase intestinal blood flow
- Splacnicectomy
Techniques to control gastric hypersecretion
- Vagotomy and pyloroplastia
- Supraselective vagotomy
Techniques to prolong intestinal transit
- Troncular vagotomy
- Reversed small bowel segment
- Reversed colon segment
- Gastric tube interpositioning
- Appendix interpositioning
- Pouches that slow down
- Recirculating loops
- Sphinters and artificial valves
- Intestinal invagination techniques
- Techniques that involve muscular sectioning or ablation
- Valves through submucosa tunneling
- Denerved intestinal segments
- Artificial periintestinal rings
- Intestinal pacemakers
- Techniques to regenerate mucosa
Techniques to avoid bacterial overgrowth
- Intestinal remodeling or enteroplastias
- Intestinal plication
- Correcting stenosis
Techniques to increase the absorption surface
- Intestinal neomucosa formation
- Techniques to prolong intestinal length
- Intestinal length elongation (Bianchi technique)
- Sequential intestinal elongation
- Intestinal elongation with mechanical distraction
- Transverse intestinal elongation (Kimura technique)
- Serial transverse enteroplasty (STEP technique)
- Intestinal pouch with an inflatable silicone implantation
Techniques to enlarge the absorption surface and to prolong transit time
- Intestine transplantation

Because of PN associated comorbilities, the initial goal in managing patients with intestinal failure is to enable PN weaning. Autologous gastrointestinal reconstruction (AGIR) further facilitates the adaptation process and attempts to reverse PN complications. The principle of AGIR relies on bowel dilatation resulting from post-resectional adaptation and the ability to manipulate this dilated bowel surgically to improve dysmotility and absorption, which thus facilitates enteral autonomy. Of the several reconstruction methods followed, tapening enteroplasty, Bianchi´s longitudinal intestinal lengthening and tailoring (LILT) and serial transverse enteroplasty (STEP) have been more widely accepted. It is now well accepted that the probability of permanent PN dependency is fairly high with remnant bowel length <40 cm. In such cases, where the chance of spontaneous adaptation is minimal, the creation of controlled obstruction to actively generate bowel dilatation is suggested with a view to performing AGIR surgery later.

Different AGIR options must be tailored individually according to the length and type of residual intestine, but the combination of various techniques may prove beneficial in certain situations than a single procedure.

An antiperistaltique bowel loop, creates partial mechanical obstruction and delays myoelectric activity --in the distal segment, which slows transit to enhance nutrient absorption [74, 75]. Reversed segment lengths of 10-15 cm for adults and around 3 cm for children have been suggested to provide maximum benefits, but establishing the ideal length and location of the reversed bowel segment remains uncertain and produces variable results when clinically applied; e.g., this technique cannot be used when the remnant bowel is <25 cm [90]. For patients with rapid intestinal transit and who do not present bowel dilation, small bowel segmental reversal may cut PN requirements [90-93].

In the event of an oversmall remnant bowel precluding AGIR, isoperistaltic colon interposition can prove a useful technique in patients with ultra SBS. In exceptional circumstances, the colon play a key role, similarly to those of the remaining small bowel.

Tapering enteroplasty, which involves excising a wedge of the antimesenteric border of the dilated bowel, followed by suturing the remnant bowel into a tube, reduces the diameter of the dilated bowel and facilitates an early return of effective peristalsis.

The intestinal plication technique was designed by the circumferencial plication of the dilated bowel after folding the redundant antimesenteric wall into the lumen to advoid a long anastomotic suture line of enteroplasty, and to also preserve the mucosal mass, which is a relevant aspect in SBS.

Revolution in SBS management came when Bianchi reported the longitudinal intestinal lengthening procedure, which doubled the length of the original segment [77], and with posterior procedure modifications.

For LILT and STEP, failure to achieve intestinal autonomy by conservative therapy is the main indication, and end-stage liver disease is the main contraindication. A sufficiently dilated intestinal segment is a common anatomical precondition for both procedures. STEP can be performed on shorter intestinal segments, and also on intricate segments such as the duodenum, which is technically not feasible by LILT. Both procedures offe a similar extent of intestinal lengthening (approximately 70%) and results in improved enteral nutrition and the reversal of PN complications. For carefully selected patients with rapid intestinal transit and a dilated bowel, LILT and STEP procedures may prove beneficial [90, 93]. Outcomes following STEP and LILT are generally similar, and the choice between these procedures may depend on the surgeon´s preference. From the technical perspective, STEP offers clear advantages over LILT as it is easily reproducible, and, above all, it can be performed primarily or repeatedly in patients who develop bowel redilation after a LILT or STEP procedure. STEP appears to have lower mortality and overall progression to transplantation rates. In children, STEP and LILT are both accepted procedures for non-transplant surgical SBS management.

Table 6. Indications for intestine transplantation

Criteria: 1. Irreversible intestinal failure has been demonstrated 2. Development of serious complications in administering parenteral nutrition. As indications, the following are acceptable: • Irreversible liver damage related to administering parenteral nutrition • Loss of deep vein accesses through thrombosis • Serious sepsis related with using deep vein catheters • Intestinal failure that usually leads to early death, despite optimum nutritional support Exclusion criteria do not differ from those normally adopted in other solid organ transplantations and can be grouped into absolute and relative.

The major revolution to occur in intestinal transplantation came when the Center for Medicare and Medical Services (USA) accepted bowel transplantation as the standard case for intestinal failure patients with failing

PN and other medical or surgical rehabilitation attempts, and it offered insurance coverage for this procedure [94].

Intestinal transplantation is a curative alternative for patients in whom intestinal rehabilitation attemps have failed and who are at risk of life-threatening PN complications [93] (Table 5). The main goal of intestinal transplantation is to restore enteral nutrition. Intestinal transplantation has several variants depending on other concomitant organ failures, which need simultaneous replacement with intestines: isolated intestinal transplantation is indicated in irreversible intestinal failure in the absence of associated severe liver dysfunction, as proven by a liver biopsy; a combined liver-intestine transplantation is indicated when intestinal failure patients have co-existing irreversible liver disease; multivisceral transplantation involves the removal and replacement of both native foregut and midgut. In this case, the graft may include liver, kidneys, and the large intestine, depending on the needs in each case. In all these transplantations, enterostomy of the distal graft ileum is performed to serve for graft surveillance through repeated biopsies made to assess allograft rejection [90]. Although intestinal transplantation is potentially life-saving for SBS, it should be reserved for patients with failed AGIR or for those who have no autologous enteral autonomy prospects [95, 96].

REFERENCES

[1] O´Keefe, Stephen J, Buchman, Alan L, Fishbein, Thomas M, Jeejeebhoy, Khursheed N, Jeppesen, Palle Bekker, Shaffer, Jonathan (2006): Short bowel syndrome and intestinal failure: consensus definition and overview. *Clinical Gastroenterol Hepatol* 4:6-10.

[2] Wilmore, Douglas W, Robinson, Malcolm K (2000): Short bowel syndrome. *World J Surg* 24:1486-1492.

[3] Ballesteros Pomar, M. D, Vidal Casariego, A: (2007): Síndrome de intestino corto: definición, causas, adaptación intestinal y sobrecrecimiento bacteriano. *Nutr Hosp* 22 (Supl. 2):74-85.

[4] Thompson, Jon S (2014): Short bowel syndrome and malabsorption - causes and prevention. *Viszeralmedicine* 30:174-178.

[5] Thompson, Jon S, Rochling, Fedja A, Weseman, Rebecca A, Mercer, David F (2010): Current management of short bowel syndrome. *Current Probl Surg* 49:52-115.

[6] Dabney, Anne, Thompson, Jon, Di Baise, John, Sudan, Debra, McBridge, Corrigan (2004): Short bowel syndrome after trauma. *Am J Surg* 188:792-795.

[7] Amiot, Aurelien, Messing, Bernard, Corcos, Olivier, Panis, Yves, Joly, Francisca (2013): Determinants of home parenteral nutrition dependency and survival of 268 patients with non-malignant short bowel syndrome. *Clin Nutr* 32:368-374.

[8] DiBaise, John K, Parrish, Carol Rees (2014): Short bowel syndrome in adults-Part 1 Physiological alterations and clinical consequences. *Practical Gastroenterology* 132:30-39.

[9] Thompson Jon S (2000): Comparison of massive vs. repeated resection leading to short bowel syndrome. *J Gastrointest Surg* 4:101-104.

[10] Thompson, Jon S, Langnas, Alan N, Pinch, Lewis W, Kaufman, Stuart, Quingley, Eamonn M, Vanderhoof, Jon A (1995): Surgical approach to short-bowel syndrome. Experience in a population of 160 patients. *Ann Surg* 222:600-607.

[11] Scolapio, James S, Fleming, C Richard, Kelly, Darlene G,, Wick, Dawn M, Zinsmeister, Alan R (1999): Survival of home parenteral nutrition treated patients: 20 years of experience at the Mayo Clinic. *Mayo Clin Proc* 74:217-222.

[12] Messing, Bernard, Lémann, Marc, Landais, Paul, Gouttebel, Marie-Claude, Boncompain, Michèl Gérard, Saudin, François, Vangossum, André, Beau, Philippe, Guédon, Claire, Barnoud, Didier, Beliah, Martine, Joyeux, Henri, Bouletreau, Paul, Carpentier, Yvon, Rambaud, Jean-Claude (1995): Prognosis of patients with nonmalignat chronic intestinal failure receiving long-term home parenteral nutrition. *Gastroenterology* 108:1005-1010.

[13] Carbonnel, Frank, Cosnes, Jacques, Chevret, Sylvie, Beaugerie, Laurent, Ngo, Yann, Malafosse, Michel, Parc, Rolland, Le Quintrec, Ives, Gendre, Jean Pièrre (1996): The role of anatomic factors in nutritional autonomy after extensive small bowel resection. *J Parenter Enteral Nutr* 20:275-280.

[14] Scolapio, James S, Fleming, C. Richard (1998): Short bowel syndrome. *Gastroenterol Clin North Am* 27:467-479.

[15] Nightingale, Jeremy M. D., Bartran, Clives L, Lennard-Jones, John E (1991): Lenght of residual small bowel after partial resection: correlation between radiographic and surgical measurement. *Gastrointestinal Radiol* 16:305-306.

[16] Buchman, Alan L, Scolapio, James, Fryer, Jon (2003): AGA Technical Review on short bowel syndrome and intestinal transplantation. *Gastroenterology* 124:1111-1134.

[17] Jeejeebhoy, Kursheed N (2002): Short bowel syndrome: a nutritional and medical approach *CMAJ* 166:1297-1302.

[18] Ninghtingale, Jeremy N. D. (2001): Management of patients with a short bowel. *World J Gastroenterol* 7:741-751.

[19] Thompson, Jon S, Ferguson, Debra C (2000): Effect of the distal remnant on ileal adaptation. *J Gastroenterol Surg* 4:430-434.

[20] American Gastroenterological Association (2003). Short bowel syndrome and intestinal transplantation: medical position statement. 124:1105-1110.

[21] Banerje A, Warwicker P (2002): Acute renal failure and metabolic disturbances in the short bowel syndrome. *Q J Med* 95:37-40.

[22] Cavicchi, Maryan, Beau, Philippe, Crenn, Pascal, Degott, Claude, Messing, Bernard (2000): Prevalence of liver disease and contributing factors in patients receiving home parenteral nutrition for permanent intestinal failure. *Ann Intern Med* 132:525-532.

[23] Messing, Bernard, Crenn, Pascal, Beau, Philippe, Boutron-Ruault, Christine, Rambaud, Jean- Claude, Matuchansky, Claude (1999): Long-term survival and parenteral nutrition dependence in adult patients with the short bowel syndrome. *Gastroenterology* 117:1043-1050.

[24] Nordgaard, Inge, Hansen, Birthen S, Mortensen, Per B (1996): Importance od colonic support for energy absorption as small bowel failure proceeds. *Am J Clin Nutr* 64:222-231.

[25] Jeppesen PB, Mortensen PB (2000): Intestinal failure defined by measurement of intestinal energy and weight absorption. *Gut* 46:701-706.

[26] Crenn, Pascal, Vahedi, Kouroche, Lavergne-Slove, Anne, Cynober, Luc, Matuchansky, Claude, Messing, Bernard (2003): Plasma citrulline: a marker of enterocyte mass in villous atrophy-associated small bowel disease. *Gastroenterology* 124:1210-1219.

[27] Crenn, Pascal, Messing, Bernard, Cynober, Luc (2008): Citrulline as a biomarker of intestinal failure due to enterocyte mass reduction. *Clin Nutr* 27:328-339.

[28] Fich, Alexander, Steadman, Charles J, Phillips, Sidney F, Camilleri, Michael, Brown, Manuel L, Haddad, Anne C, Thomnforde, George M (1992): Ileocolonic transit does not change after right hemicolectomy. *Gastroenterology* 103:794-799.

[29] Petersen, Craig (2005): D-lactic acidosis. *Nutr Clin Pract* 20:634-645.

[30] Miguel E de, Gómez de Segura I, Bonet H, Rodríguez Montes, JA, Mata A (1994): Trophyc effects of neurotensin in massive small bowel intestin in the rat. *Dig Dis Sci* 39:65-68.

[31] Gomez de Segura I, de Miguel E, Mata A, Rodríguez Montes JA (1994): Plasma enteroglucagon levels in different models of intestinal resection in the rat. *Dig Dis Sci* 39:59-64.

[32] Dowling, R Herman (1973): Intestinal adaptation. *N Engl J Med* 288:520-521.

[33] Rodríguez Montes, J. A., Murillo Taravillo A, Galera Davidson H, Arcelus Imaz IM (1975): Cambios morfológicos en el intestino después de la resección. Estudio experimental. *Cir Esp* 29:29-34. Wilmore, Douglas W, Byrne, Theresa A, Persinger, Rebecca L (1997): Short bowel syndrome: new therapeutic approaches. *Curr Probl Surg* 34:389-444.

[34] Cisler, Jason J, Buchman, Alan L (2005): Intestinal adaptation in shorth bowel syndrome. J Investig Med 53:402-413.

[35] Tappenden, Kelly A (2014): Intestinal adaptation following resection. J *Parent Ent Nutr* 38 (Suppl 1): 23S-31S.

[36] Spencer, Ariel U, Kovacevich, Debra, McKinney-Barnett, Michelle, Hair, Deanna, Canham, Julie, Maksym Christopher, Teitelbaum, Daniel H (2008): Pediatric short-bowel syndrome: the cost of comprehensive care. *Am J Clin Nutr* 2008; 88:1552-1559.

[37] Thompson, Jon S, Quigley, Eamonn MM, Adrian, Thomas E (1999): Factors affecting outcome following proximal and distal intestinal resection in the dog: an examination of the relative roles of mucosal adaptation, motility, luminal factors, and enteric peptides. *Dig Dis Sci* 44:63-74.

[38] Schmidt T, Pfeiffer A, Hackelsberger N, Widmer R, Meisel C, Kaess H (1996): Effect of intestinal resection on human small bowel motility. *Gut* 38: 859-863.

[39] Soden, Jason S (2010): Clinical assessment of the child with intestinal failure. *Semin Pediatr Surg* 19:10-19.

[40] Shiomi, Masaya, Wakabayashi, Yoshikuyi, Sano, Tsuyoshi, Shinoda, Yuichi, Nimura, Yuji, Ishimura, Yuzuru, Suematsu, Makoto (1998): Nitric oxide suppression reversibly attenuates mitochondrial dysfunction and cholestasis in endotoxemic rat liver. *Hepatology* 27: 108-115.

[41] Cole, Conrad R, Ziegler, Thomas R (2007): Small bowel bacterial overgrowth: a negative factor in gut adaptation in pediatric SBS. *Curr Gastroenterol Rep* 9:456-462.

[42] Thompson Jon S, Rochling, Fedja A, Weseman, Rebecca, Mercer, David F (2011): Current management of the short bowel syndrome. *Surg Clin North Am* 91:493-510.

[43] Davidovics, Zev H, Carter, Beth A, Luna, Ruth A, Hollister, Emily B, Shulman, Robert I, Versalovic, James (2015): The fecal microbiome in pediatric patients with short bowel syndrome. *JPEN* doi:10.1177/0148607115591216.

[44] Alpers, David H, Stenson, William F (1996): Does total parenteral nutrition-induced intestinal mucosal atrophy occur in humans and can it be affected by enteral supplements? *Curr Opin Gastroenterol* 12:169-173.

[45] Buchnman, Alan L, Moukarzel, Adib A (1995): Parenteral nutrition is associated with intestinal morphologic and functional changes in humans. *J Parent Ent Nutr* 19:453-460.

[46] Scolapio, James S, Camilleri, Michael, Fleming, Richard C, Oenning, La Vonne, Burton, Duane D, Sebo, Thomas J, Batts, Kenneth P (1997): Effect of growth hormone, glutamine and diet adaptation in short bowel syndrome: a randomized, controlled study. *Gastroenterology* 113:1074-1081.

[47] Platell, Cameron F. E., Coster, Jane, McCauley, Rosalie D, Hall, John C (2002): The management of patients with the short bowel syndrome. *World J Gastroenterol* 8:13-20.

[48] Matarese, Laura, Seidner, Douglas L, Steiger, Ezra (2004): Growth hormone, glutamine, and modified diet for intestinal adaptation. *J Acad Nutr Diet* 104:1265-1272.

[49] Alpers, David H (2006): Glutamine: do the data support the cause for glutamine supplementation in humans? *Gastroenetrology* 130:S106-S116.

[50] Drozdowski, Laurie, Thomson, Alan BR (2006): Intestinal mucosal adaptation. *World J Gastroenterol* 12:4614-4627.

[51] Martin GR, Beck PL, Sigalet DL (2006): Gut hormones, and short bowel syndrome: the enigmatic role of glucagon-like peptide-2 in the regulation of intestinal adaptation. *World J Gastroenterol* 12:4117-4129.

[52] Jeppesen PB, Sanguinetti EL, Buchman A, Howard L, Scolapio JS, Ziegler TR, Gregory J, Tappenden KA, Holst J, Mortensen PB (2005): Teduglutide (ALX-0600), a dipeptidyl peptidase IV resistant glucagon-

like peptide 2 analogue, improves intestinal function in short bowel syndrome patients. *Gut* 54:1224-1231.

[53] Jeppesen, Palle Bekker (2012): Teduglutide, a novel glucagon-like peptide 2 analog, in the treatment of patients with short bowel syndrome. *Therap Adv Gastroenterol* 5:159-171.

[54] Krsek M, Rosicksa M, Haluzik M, Svobodova J, Kotrlikova E, Jistova V, Lacinoca Z, Jarkovska Z (2002): Plasma ghrelin levels in patients with short bowel syndrome. *Endocr Res* 28:27-33.

[55] Rodríguez Montes JA, Spreaffico J Mª, Carmena A, Díaz-Florez L, Arcelus I (1976): Cambios en la mucosa gástrica en perros con resección intestinal. Estudio óptico y ultraestructural. *Rev Esp Enf Ap Digest* 4:673-682.

[56] O´Keefe, Stephen J (2006): Bacterial overgrowth and liver complications in short bowel intestinal failure patients. *Gastroenterology* 130:S67-S69.

[57] Matarese, Laura E, Seidner, Douglas L, Steiger, Ezra (2003): The role of probiotic in gastrointestinal disease. *Nutr Clin Pract* 18:507-516.

[58] Rodríguez-Montes, José Antonio (2014): Intestino corto: de la resección al trasplante. *Nutr Hosp* 30:961-966.

[59] Jeppesen, Palle Bekker (2014): Spectrum of short bowel syndrome in adults: intestinal insufficiency to intestinal failure. *J Parent Ent Nutr* 38 (1 Suppl): 8S-13S.

[60] Storch, Kenneth J (2014): Overview of short bowel syndrome: clinical features, pathophysiology, impact, and management. *J Parent Ent Nutr* 3 (1 Suppl):5S-7S.

[61] Nightingale, Jeremy N (2003): Hepatobiliary, renal and bone complications of intestinal failure. *Best Pract Res Clin Gastroenterol* 17:907-929.

[62] Rodríguez Montes, J. A. (1979): Trastornos psiquiátricos consecutivos a resección intestinal masiva. *Rev Clin Esp* 152: 153-154.

[63] Thompson, Jon S (1996): The role of prophylactic cholecystectomy in the short bowel syndrome. *Arch Surg* 131:556-559.

[64] Kelly, Darlene G, Tappenden, Kelly A, Winkler, Marlon F (2014): Short bowel syndrome: highlights of patient management, quality of life, and survival. *J Parent Ent Nutr* 38:427-437.

[65] Jeppesen, Palle Bekker (2014): Pharmacologic options for intestinal rehabilitation in patients with short bowel syndrome. *J Parent Ent Nutr* 38 (1 Suppl): 45S-52S.

[66] Secretaría de Salud (2013). Guía de Práctica Clínica: síndrome de intestino corto. Tratamiento médico-nutricional. México.

[67] Stringer, Mark D, Puntis, John W (1995): Short bowel syndrome. *Arch Dis Child* 73:170-173.

[68] Devine, Richard M, Kelly, Kimberly A (1989): Surgical therapy of the short bowel syndrome. *Gastroenterol Clin North Am* 18:603-618.

[69] Rodríguez Montes JA (1990): Tratamiento del intestino corto. An R Acad Nac Med (Madrid) 107:91-113.

[70] Mackby, M Judson, Richards, Victor, Gilfillan, Rutherford S, Florindia, Rosario (1965): Methods of increasing the efficiency of residual small bowel segments. *Am J Surg* 109:32-38.

[71] Rodríguez Montes JA, Murillo Taravillo A, Arcelus Imaz IMª (1980): Un intento de recirculación intestinal en perros con resección. *Rev Esp Enf Ap Digest* 57:149-156.

[72] Hammer, John M, Seay, Patrick H, Johnston, Richard L, Hill, Edward J, Prust, Frank H, Campbell, Ruth J (1959): The effect of antiperistaltic bowel segment and intestinal emptying time. *Arch Surg* 79:537-554.

[73] Kumao, Sako, Blackman, George E (1962: The use of a reversed jejunal segment after massive resection of the small bowel. *Am J Surg* 103:202-205.

[74] Rodríguez Montes JA, Galera Davidson H, Murillo taravillo A, Arcelus Imaz IMª (1975): Bases experimentales para el empleo de asas antiperistalticas en cirugía intestinal. *Rev Quir Esp* 2:236-241.

[75] Rodríguez Montes JA, Murillo Taravillo A, Arcelus IMª (1976): Effects d´une anse antiperistaltique après resection gastrointestinale (Lèttre). *Nouv Prèsse Méd* 5:2548.

[76] Shepard, Duncan (1966): Antiperistaltic bowel segment in the treatment of the short bowel syndrome. *Ann Surg* 163:850-855.

[77] Bianchi A (1980): Intestinal loop lengthening -a technique for increasing small intestinal length. *J Pediatr Surg* 15:145-151.

[78] Rodríguez Montes JA, Murillo Taravillo A, Arcelus Imaz IMª (1978): Implantación de anillos periintestinales en perros con intestino corto. *Rev Esp Enf Ap Digest* 54:41-50.

[79] Hutcher, Neil E, Salzberg, Arnold M (1971): Preileal transposition of colon to prevent the development of short bowel syndrome in puppies with 90 percent small intestinal resection. *Surgery* 70:189-197.

[80] Pigot, François, Messing, Bernard, Chaussade, Stanislas, Pfeiffer, Albrecht, Pouliquen, Xavier, Jian, Raymond (1990): Severe short bowel

syndrome with a surgically reversed small bowel segment. *Dig Dis Sci* 35:137-144.

[81] Garcia, Victor F, Templeton, John M, Eichelberger, Martin R, Koop, Everett C, Vinograd, Itzak (1981): Colon interposistion for the short bowel syndrome. *J Pediatr Surg* 16:994-995.

[82] Glick, Philip L, de Lorimier, Alfred A, Adzick, N Scott, Harrison, Michael R (1984): Colon interposition: an adjuvant operation for short-gut syndrome. *J Pediatr Surg* 19:719-725.

[83] Bianchi A (1984): Intestinal lengthening: an experimental and clinical review. *J R Soc Med* 77 (suppl 3):35-41.

[84] Kimura, Ken, Soper, Robert T (1993): A new bowel elongation technique for the short bowel syndrome using the isolated bowel segment iowa models. *J Pediatr Surg* 28:792-794.

[85] Thompson, Jon S (1987): Growth of neomucosa after intestinal resection. *Arch Surg* 122:316-319.

[86] Pappis Ch, Kairis MZ, Willital GH (1986): Enterization of the dural patch. An experimental study. *Pediatr Surg Int* 1:192-196.

[87] Fisher, Jeremy, Sparks, Eric A, Khan, Faraz A, Dionigi, Beatrice, Wu, Hao, Brazzo, Joseph III, Fauza, Dario, Modi, Biren, Safranski, David L, Jaksic, Tom (2015): Extraluminal distraction enterogenesis using shape-memory polymer. *J Pediatric Surg* 50:938-942.

[88] Pahari, Mohan P, Brown, Melissa L, Elias, Georg, Nseir, Hannan, Banner, Barbara Rastellini, Cristiana, Cicalese, Luca (2007): Development of a bioartificial new intestinal segment using an acellular matrix scaffold. *Gut* 56:585-586.

[89] Layzell, Trevor, Collin, Jack (1981): Retrograde electrical pacing of the small intestine -a new treatment for the short bowel syndrome. *Br J Surg* 68: 711-713.

[90] Rege, Aparna (2014): The surgical approach to short bowel syndrome-autologous reconstruction versus transplantation. *Visceralmedizin* 30:179-189.

[91] Beyer-Berjot, Laura, Joly, Francisca, Maggiori, Leon, Corcos, Olivier, Bouhnik, Yoram, Bretagnol, Frédérick, Panis, Ives (2012): Segmental reversal of the small bowel can end permanent parenteral nutrition dependency: an experience of 38 adults with short bowel syndrome. A*nn Surg* 256:739-44; discussion 744-45.

[92] Iyer, Kishore R (2014): Surgical management of short bowel syndrome. *J Parent Ent Nutr* 38:53S-59S.

[93] Frongia, Giovanni, Kessler, Markus, Weih, Sandra, Nickkholg, Arash, Merhabi, Arianeb, Hollanz-Cunz, Stephan (2013): Comparison of LILT and STEP procedures in children with short bowel syndrome -a systematic review of the literature. *J Pediatr Surg* 48:1794-1805.
[94] Centers for Medicare and Medicaid Services: Medicare Coverage Policy Decisions (2000): Intestinal and Multivisceral Transplantation. CAG-00036. October, 4.
[95] Rege, Aparna (2013): Autologous gastrointestinal reconstruction: review of optimal nontransplant surgical option for adults and children with short bowel syndrome. *Nutr Clin Pract* 28:65-74.
[96] Sudan, D (2014): The current state of intestine transplantation: indications, techniques, outcomes and challenges. *Am J Transpl* 14:1976-1984.

BIOGRAPHICAL SKETCHES

Jose Antonio Rodriguez-Montes, MD

Affiliation:

- Professor of Surgery, *Universidad Autónoma de Madrid*, Spain
- Chief. *Servicio de Cirugía General y del Aparato Digestivo, Hospital Universitario "La Paz,"* Madrid, Spain

Date of Birth: 04-04-1945

Education:

- Graduated in 1971 and Doctorated in 1975 (*cum laude* and *Extraordinary Doctoral Award*) at *Facultad de Medicina* of the *Universidad de Granada*, Spain. Diplomed in Nutrition at School of Nutrition of same University.
- Specialisation in General and Digestive Surgery at Department of Surgery of the *Hospital Universitario de Granada*, Spain, between 1971-75.
- Postdoctoral Research Fellow at the Physiological Laboratory of Cambridge University (UK) between 1975 and 1976, and Fellow Visitor at Department of Surgery of same University in 1978 (Scholarship from *Ministerio de Educación y Ciencia* of Spain, The British Council and The Wellcome Trust Foundation).

- *Medecin Resident Etranger* at *Service de Chirurgie Général, Digestive et Vascular* of the *Hôpital Ambroise Paré* of Paris (France), between 1980-81 (Scholarship from *Collège de Médecine de Hôpitaux de Paris*)

Address:
Servicio de Cirugía General y del Aparato Digestivo
Hospital Universitario "La Paz", 5ª planta
Paseo de la Castellana, 261
28035 Madrid. Spain
email:ja.rodriguezmontes@uam.es
email: rodriguezmontes@gmail.com

Research and Professional Experience:

- Active in the scientific research, was involved a principal investigator in several national and international projects research. Autor/coauthor of more 260 published manuscripts, more of the half of whom on peer-review journals wit Impact Factor. Editor of 16 published books, author/coauthor of 110 book chapters and of more 550 contributions to national, international, European and world congresses. He has been Director of more of 90 doctoral thesis, and 25 projects research granted by national and international scientific and medical institutions.
-Professor Rodríguez-Montes focusing his research on the emergency surgery, short bowel syndrome, conservative splenic surgery, biliary prothesis, colorectal cancer surgery, and others. He was awarded Spanish awards for research and academy activities.
- Expert/Evaluator and Advisor of several national and international research and medical institutions.
- Past President of the *Sociedad Española de Investigaciones Quirúrgicas.*

Professional Appointments:

- Since 1977 he is surgeon staff of the *Hospital Universitario "La Paz"* at Madrid (Spain); has been Chief of the *Servicio de Cirugía Experimental*, Chief of *Servicio de Cirugía General y del Apararo Digestivo*, and Vice-Director of Research and Teaching of same hospital.
- Between 1984 and 1996 he was Lecturer in Surgery and since 1996 to 2015 he has been Full Professor of Surgery of the *Universidad Autonoma de Madrid*; between 1990 and 2005 was involved as Chairman of Department of Surgery, and between 2007 and 2011 was involved as Dean of the

Medecine Faculty of same University. Since the end 2015 he is Emeritus Professor of Surgery of the Universidad Autónoma de Madrid.

Honors:

- He is Member of top several academic institutions of Spain and Honorary Member of cientific societies (*Sociedad Española de Investigaciones Quirúrgicas, Sociedad Ibero-Latino-Americana de Cirujanos, Sociedad Cubana de Cirugía, Colegio Brasileiro de Cirurgia,* and others).
- Permanent Member of the *Real Academia de Doctores de España* (Medicine Section)
- Corresponding Academic of the *Real Academia Nacional de Medicina*, and *Real Academia Nacional de Farmacia* (Spain)
- Corresponding Honorary Member of the *Real Academia de Medicina y Cirugía de Valladolid* and of the *Real Academia de Medicina de Andalucía Oriental* (Spain)
- Corresponding Academic of the *Real Academia de Medicina de Sevilla*, *Real Academia de Medicina del Principado de Asturias*, *Real Academia de Medicina de Murcia*, *Real Academia de Medicina del País Vasco*, *Real Academia de Medicina de la Comunidad Valenciana* and the *Real Academia de Medicina de Canarias.*
- Gold Medal of the *Universidad de Castilla-La Mancha* (Spain).
- Gold Master of the *Real Forum de Alta Dirección* (Spain).
- Member of Merit of the *Fundación Carlos III* (Spain).
- Member of the International College of Surgeons, British Surgical Research, Collegium Internationale de Chirurgiae Digestivae, Association Française de Chirurgie, Asociación Mexicana de Gastroenterología, Societé Internationale de Chirurgie, The Academy of Surgical Research (USA), and others.
- Visiting Professor of several universities and institutions: Bolonia, *La Habana*, Paris, Universidade Federal do Rio Grande do Sul (Brasil). Hüddinge University Hospital (Sweden) and others.
- Guest Speaker of international congresses and events celebrated in Madrid, Barcelona, Bolonia, Paris, Fortaleza (Brasil), *La Habana* (Cuba), Rio Grande do Sul (Brasil), Damascus (Syria), Moscow (Russia) and others.

Publications Last Three Years:

- Menéndez P, Villarejo P, Padilla D, Menéndez JM, Rodríguez Montes JA: Diagnostic and Pronostic Significance of Serum Micrornas in Colorectal Cancer. *J Surg Oncol* 2013;107:217-220
- Menéndez P, Villarejo P, Padilla D, Menéndez JM, Rodríguez Montes JA: Marcadores Tumorales en el Cancer Colorrectal. *Cir Cir* (México) 2013; 81:169-175
- Menéndez P, Villarejo P, Padilla D, Menéndez JM, Rodríguez Montes JA: Utilidad de la Determinacion Serica del Microarna-21 en la Patologia Inflamatoria Del Colon. *Rev Gastroenterología de México* 2013;78:70-74
- Menéndez P, Villarejo P, Padilla D, Menéndez JM, Rodríguez Montes JA: Implications of the Histological Determination of *microRNAs* in the Screening, Diagnosis and Prognosis of Colorectal Cancer. *J Surg Oncol* 2013;108:70-73
- García de Lorenzo A, Rodríguez Montes JA: Metabolismo en el Ayuno Y la Agresión. Su Papel en el Desarrollo de la Desnutrición Relacionada con la Enfermedad. *Nutr Hosp Suplementos* 2013;6:1-9
- Menéndez P, Padilla D, Villarejo P, Menéndez JM, Rodríguez Montes JA: Pronostic Implications of Serum *microRNA-21* in Colorectal Cancer. *J Surg Oncol* 2013; 108:369-373
- Salinas J, Georgiev T, González-Sánchez JA, López-Ruiz E, Rodríguez Montes JA: Gastric Necrosis: A Late Complication of Nissen Fundoplication. *World J Gastrointest Surg* 2014,6:183-186
- Rombolá C, Genovés M, Tárraga P, Honguero A, León P, Triviño A, Rodríguez Montes JA: Video-Assisted Minithoracotomy Diaphragmatic Plication: Respiratory Effects in Adults. *Thorac Cardiovasc Surg* 2014;1-7
- Rodríguez-Montes JA: Intestino Corto: de la Reseccion al Trasplante. *Nutr Hosp* 2014; 30:961-968
- Rodríguez Montes JA, Menéndez P: *PAPEL DE LOS microRNA EN EL CRIBADO DEL CANCER COLORRECTAL.* Cir Esp 2014; 92:654-658
- Prieto I, Pérez-Robledo JP, Díaz San-Andrés B, Nistal M, Rodríguez Montes JA: Inflammatory Pseudotumor of the Spleen Associated with Splenic Tuberculosis. *World J Gastrointest Surg* 2014;6:248-252
- Rodríguez Montes JA, et al: Linfangioma Esplenico: Un Tumor Raro. Aportacion de Tres Casos y Revision de la Bibliografia. *Cirugía y Cirujanos* 2015. http://dx.doi.org/10.1016/ j.circir.2015.06.016.
- Cantero R, Rubio-Pérez I, León M, Alvarez M, Díaz B, Herrera A, Díaz-Domínguez J, Rodríguez Montes JA: Negative Pressure Therapy to

Reduce the Risk of Wound Infection Following Diverting Loop Ileostomy Reversal. An Initial Study. *Adv Skin and Wound Care* 2015 (in press).

Juan Solera Albero, MD, PhD

Affiliation: Coordinator Primary Care Medical Albacete z.7, Albacete, Spain

Date of Birth: 16-03-1956

Address: C/Pedro Coca. Albacete. Spain

Research and Professional Experience:

- Family doctor for 26 years experience.
- Honorary Professor Universidad Autónoma de Madrid 5 years
- Associate Professor of Medicine University of Castilla-La Mancha from 5 years
- Director of 3 doctoral theses

Professional Appointments:

- Family physician for 25 years
- Coordinator Primary Care Medical Tean Albacete z.7. Albacete. Spain
- Career Level 4 on 4
- General Secretary Society of Medicine and Surgery Albacete
- General Secretary Castilian Manchego Society of Family Physicians
- Vice President of the Medical College of Albacete

Publications Last 3 Years:

- Orgaz Gallego MP, Bermejo López P, Tricio Armero MA, Abellán Alemán J, Solera Albero J, Tárraga López PJ: Metabolic syndrome and its components in spanish postmenopausal women. Nutr Hosp. 2015;32:656-66.
- López Rubio MA, Tárraga López PJ, Rodríguez Montes JA, Frías López M del C, Solera Albero J, Bermejo López P: Subclinical hypothyroidism and cardiovascular risk. Nutr Hosp. 2015; 31:2095-102
- Solera Albero J, Tárraga López PJ, Carbayo Herencia JA, López Cara MA, Celada Rodríguez A, Cerdán Oliver M, Ocaña López JM: Influence of diet and lifestyle in colorectal cancer. Rev Esp Enferm Dig. 2007; 99:190-200.

- López Cara MA, Tárraga López PJ, Cerdán Oliver M, Ocaña López JM, Celada Rodríguez A, Solera Albero J, Palomino Medina MA: Constipation in the population over 50 years of age in Albacete province. Rev Esp Enferm Dig. 2006; 98:449-59

Pedro J. Tárraga López, MD, PhD

Affiliation: Associate Professor of Medicine University of Castilla-La Mancha, Spain

Date of Birth: 17/09/1960

Education:

Address: C/Angel 53-1E. Albacete, Spain

Research and Professional Experience:
- Family doctor for 21 years experience
- Medical Director at University Hospital of Albacete 4 years. Spain
- Honorary Professor Universidad Autónoma de Madrid 15 years
- Associate Professor of Medicine University of Castilla-La Mancha from 2005 onward
- Doctoral dissertation in 1996. Extraordinary Doctoral Award
- Director of 32 doctoral theses.
- 105 doctoral tutor Thesis
- 110 Director PhD courses

Professional Appointments:
- Coordinator Primary Care Medical Tean Casas Ibanez (Albacete). Spain
- Medical Director of Primary Care Integrated Management of Albacete
- Career Level 4 on 4
- President Society of Medicine and Surgery of Albacete. Spain
- VicePresident Castilian Manchego Society of Family Physicians
- Treasurer of the Medical College of Albacete

Honors:
- PhD Prize 1996

- 12 Research Awards for contributions to Congress as Oral Communication or Poster

Publications Last 3 Years:

- Tárraga-López PJ, Celada-Rodríguez A, Cerdán-Oliver M, Solera-Albero J, Ocaña-López JM, López-Cara MA, De Miguel-Clave J: A pharmacoeconomic evaluation of statins in the treatment of hypercholesterolaemia in the primary care setting in Spain. Pharmacoeconomics. 2005;2
- Tárraga Marcos ML, Rosich N, Panisello Royo JM, Gálvez Casas A, Serrano Selva JP, Rodríguez-Montes JA, Tárraga López PJ: Efficacy of motivational interventions in the treatment of overweight and obesity. Nutr Hosp. 2014; 30:741-8
- Tárraga López PJ, Albero JS, Rodríguez-Montes JA: Primary and secondary prevention of colorectal cancer. Clin Med Insights Gastroenterol. 2014; 7:33-46.
- Tárraga López PJ, Garcia-Norro Herreros FJ, Tárraga Marcos L, Solera Albero J, González López E, Ruiz García A, Pallarés Carratalá V, Castro Navarro JL, Alins Presas J, Panisello Royo JM: Active interventions in hypercholesteroloemia patients with high cardiovascular risk in primary care. Nutr Hosp. 2015; 31:2261-8
- Tárraga López PJ, García-Norro Herreros FJ, Tárraga Marcos L, Solera Albero J, González López E, Ruiz García A, Pallarés Carratalá V, Castro Navarro JL, Alins Presas J, Panisello Royo JM: Active interventions in hypercholesteroloemia patients with high cardiovascular risk in primary care; estudio ESPROCOL. Nutr Hosp. 2015; 31:2727-34.
- Tarraga P, Orgaz M, Bermejo P, Abellan J, Tricio M, Tarraga M: Prevalence of metabolic syndrome and its components in spanish postmenopausal women. J Hypertens. 2015; 33 Suppl 1:e48
- Bermejo P, Vivo A, Tárraga PJ, Rodríguez-Montes JA: Development of Interpretable Predictive Models for BPH and Prostate Cancer. Clin Med Insights Oncol. 2015;9:15-24

In: Short Bowel Syndrome (SBS)
Editor: Violet Chapman
ISBN: 978-1-63484-944-9

Chapter 3

SURGICAL MANAGEMENT OF SHORT BOWEL SYNDROME: CURRENT INTESTINAL LENGTHENING TECHNIQUES

Chasen J. Greig and Robert A. Cowles*
Yale University School of Medicine, Yale-New Haven Hospital,
Section of Pediatric Surgery, New Haven, Connecticut, US

ABSTRACT

Intestinal failure (IF) in the pediatric population most commonly results from a congenital abnormality or major intra-abdominal catastrophe in the neonatal period or early in life. The term short bowel syndrome (SBS) is commonly used interchangeably with IF and is one of the most common causes of pediatric IF although other etiologies of IF exist despite normal or near normal bowel length. The management of both IF and SBS currently relies upon parenteral nutrition (PN), but the surgical management of SBS has undergone an extensive maturation process in the last several decades. While intestinal transplantation is now a viable option for some patients, it is still far from first line therapy and outcomes have lagged behind those of other organs. The central tenet of the currently available and emerging surgical intestinal lengthening techniques is increasing the function and absorptive capacity of the

* Corresponding author: Robert A. Cowles. E-mail: robert.cowles@yale.edu.

remaining bowel. As early as the late 19th century, animal models were used to develop viable lengthening procedures, which led to innovative procedures of the time including antiperistaltic segments, valves and intestinal pacing. These early developments spurred the evolution of techniques as surgical intervention proved effective in increasing intestinal function. More recently, the serial transverse enteroplasty (STEP) and spiral intestinal lengthening and tailoring (SILT) procedures have been developed, taking advantage of progress in understanding of bowel physiology and decades of surgical experience. This review will summarize the current state of surgical approaches to bowel lengthening, with a brief overview of pertinent historical procedures important in the progression of management of this disease.

INTRODUCTION

Of all the divisions of the gastrointestinal tract, the small bowel is the only segment which cannot be fully removed and life sustained [1]. Intestinal Failure (IF) can be defined as insufficient bowel length to provide the absorptive capacity needed to meet the metabolic demands of the body. There is, however, no clear consensus in terminology as some may require the inclusion of dependence on PN in the definition [2]. The true incidence and prevalence of the disease is not known, but an estimated 45,000 patients in the United States suffer from intestinal failure based on data collected on home PN use [3]. The etiology of IF differs between children and adults, corresponding to differences in metabolic demand; children in a state of growth and development in contrast to adults in a homeostatic state. In the pediatric population, further differences can be seen based upon socioeconomic status. In developing countries, transient factors are most commonly involved, as opposed to developed countries in which permanent factors are most common (Table 1) [2].

Current medical management of intestinal failure in the pediatric population is based upon administration of PN to not only support fluid and nutritional requirements, but to allow for effective intestinal repair and adaptation. As one might expect, PN requirements and formulations will vary with the underlying cause of IF. Medical management of IF is thus complex and requires careful consideration of risks and benefits. This represents a major challenge for those patients who are likely to require lifelong PN [4], as therapy can result in a host of serious and even fatal complications [5, 6].

Table 1. Selected Causes of Intestinal Failure

Transient	Permanent	
Infection	Primary:	Secondary:
Temporary disturbances - mechanical (e.g., obstruction) - functional (e.g., ileus)	- Mucosal Enteropathies (e.g., Microvillus Inclusion Disease, Tufting Enteropathy)	- Short Bowel Syndrome Congenital or acquired loss of intestinal length
	- Motility Disorders (e.g., Hirschprung Disease, Chronic Intestinal Pseudo-Obstruction)	

While many may see intestinal transplantation (ITx) as the natural destination for these patients, it remains far from first-line therapy in IF refractory to medical management. While the practice of ITx has made many strides in recent years, it has not yet replicated the outcomes seen in the transplantation of other organs [7, 8]. In this setting, surgical techniques for lengthening bowel and thereby increasing functional GI mass and the likelihood of enteral autonomy are of great importance. The aim of this chapter is to describe the development of intestinal lengthening techniques and to outline currently used procedures to lengthen bowel.

EARLY TECHNIQUES IN BOWEL LENGTHENING

Interest in surgical procedures that lengthen bowel dates back to the late 19th century. Early investigators in this area included Mall and Singleton, whom were important innovators in the technique of reversed intestinal segments. The observation that reversed segments retained polarity in peristalsis led to experimentation with the procedure in animal models as a means of slowing intestinal transit and increasing absorption [9]. Gibson performed one of the earliest known small intestinal reversed segments in 1962 in a human patient after massive bowel resection (Figure 1). The 84 year old patient not only survived, but went on to demonstrate weight gain and cessation of malabsorptive diarrhea in the follow-up period [10]. One of the earliest reports of reversed segments in the pediatric population was by

Warden, who employed the technique as a salvage operation for infants with short bowel syndrome following massive resection [11].

Other early techniques included recirculating loops, gastric tubes, and vagotomy; however, these failed to yield the necessary positive results to be accepted. It wasn't until Schiller described the creation of an artificial sphincter in the intestine that another novel technique gained traction alongside reversed segments. Using dogs, Schiller created a chronically constricted segment of intestine by removing the longitudinal muscle and with it the normal mechanisms by which the lumen is opened [12]. The creation of a "neosphincter" led to the development of a technique for an intestinal valve to slow transit in patients with SBS. Waddell describes the technique of jejunocolic valves created in human patients suffering from rapid transit, with reasonable initial results [13].

The commonality amongst most of these initial techniques was the intent to slow intestinal transit allowing for increased absorption for a given length of bowel. While many of these techniques in animal models and in human subjects succeeded in this goal, it was not without consequences. It was not uncommon for significant bowel obstruction to develop, sometimes even necessitating reversal of the responsible procedure. Additionally, an unforeseen complication during development of these procedures was the presence of bacterial overgrowth when intestinal transit was slowed and periods of stasis were prolonged. This represented a serious concern for infection of the critical amount of remaining bowel in these patients.

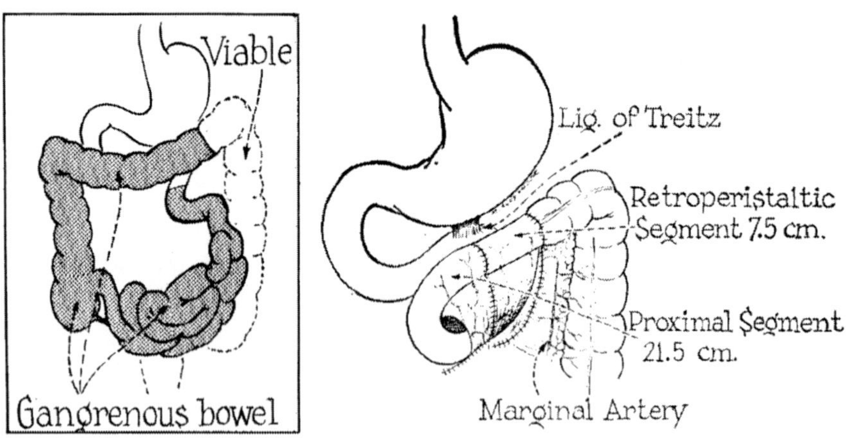

Figure 1. Original figures from Gibson et al. [10] depicting the initial insult (left) and subsequent repair with antiperistaltic segment (right).

In light of these difficulties the development of colonic interposition, initially described by Lloyd [14], was felt to represent a step foreword. The use of isoperistaltic colon interpositional segments was not associated with either obstruction or bacterial overgrowth, and initial results were promising, as reported by Glick [15]. This technique remained popular throughout the decade following its initial introduction [16-18], but eventually fell out of favor when newer techniques were developed.

THE EVOLUTION OF SURGERY TO TREAT SBS

With continued interest in non-transplant surgical techniques for SBS came further innovation in the field. At the end of the 20th century, several developments were made which would serve as the basis for our current understanding of SBS and procedures used in its treatment.

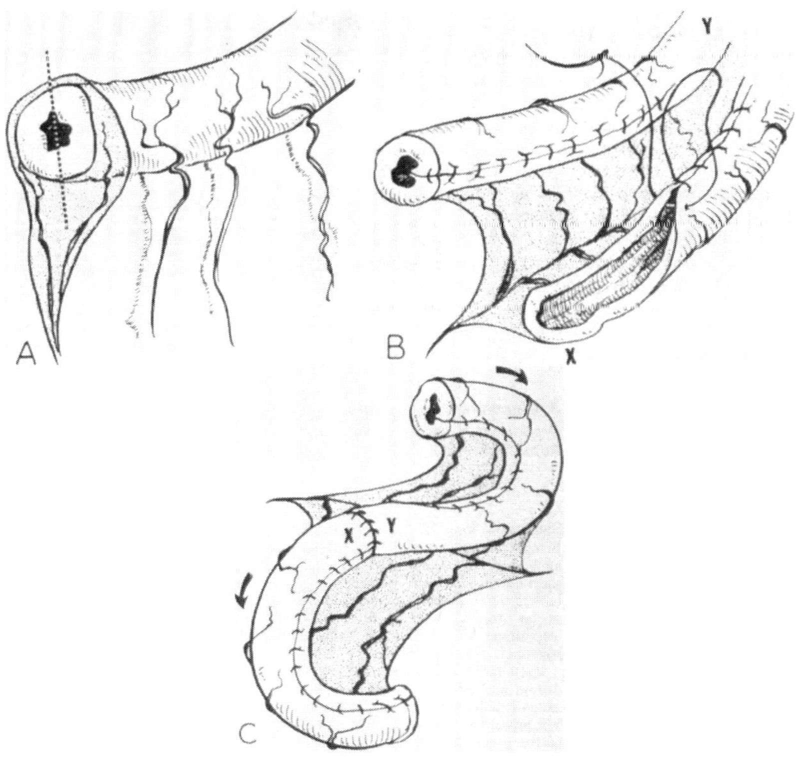

Figure 2. The Bianchi procedure or LILT [20].

Bianchi is considered a pioneer in the field of intestinal lengthening surgery. In 1980, his landmark paper described the technique of longitudinal division of dilated small bowel segments based upon separate and distinct blood supply from the mesentery (Figure 2) [19]. This technique, commonly referred to as "The Bianchi," resulted in nearly double the small bowel length per a given segment, but required significant handling of the mesentery and tedious dissection. Despite this, results were encouraging and the procedure gained popularity over the next decade [20]. Throughout this time the procedure underwent a few minor modifications and eventually became known as longitudinal intestinal lengthening and tailoring (LILT). Bianchi and others performing the procedure began publishing long-term outcomes in the mid-1990's [21-26] which established LILT as one of the primary lengthening techniques in the management of SBS.

In 1993, Kimura described his technique for intestinal elongation by taking advantage of the principle of collateral formation. His observation that the remaining small bowel segment in SBS is often substantially dilated prompted him to devise approaches which could utilize this dilatation. Additionally, he aimed to minimize the mesenteric manipulation and difficult technical aspect of the Bianchi procedure. What developed was a staged procedure in which the dilated small bowel undergoes seromyotomy to expose the mucosa, which is then fixed to a "donor" organ such as the liver or abdominal wall. Following an interval of 8-10 weeks during which collaterals are formed, the patient returns to the OR where the dilated and now dual-perfused intestine is split longitudinally, and subsequently re-anastomosed end-to-end (Figure 3) [27]. This provided nearly double the length of the small bowel and preserved the muscular orientation for peristalsis, while minimizing the manipulation of the mesentery.

Georgeson and his colleagues were amongst the leaders in improvement of the management of children with SBS [28], which led to his contributions to the surgical lengthening techniques. He and his group developed a staged procedure utilizing the previously described creation of artificial valves to induce small bowel dilatation and adaptation, followed by a lengthening technique [29]. The techniques used for the second stage included those described by Kimura and Bianchi.

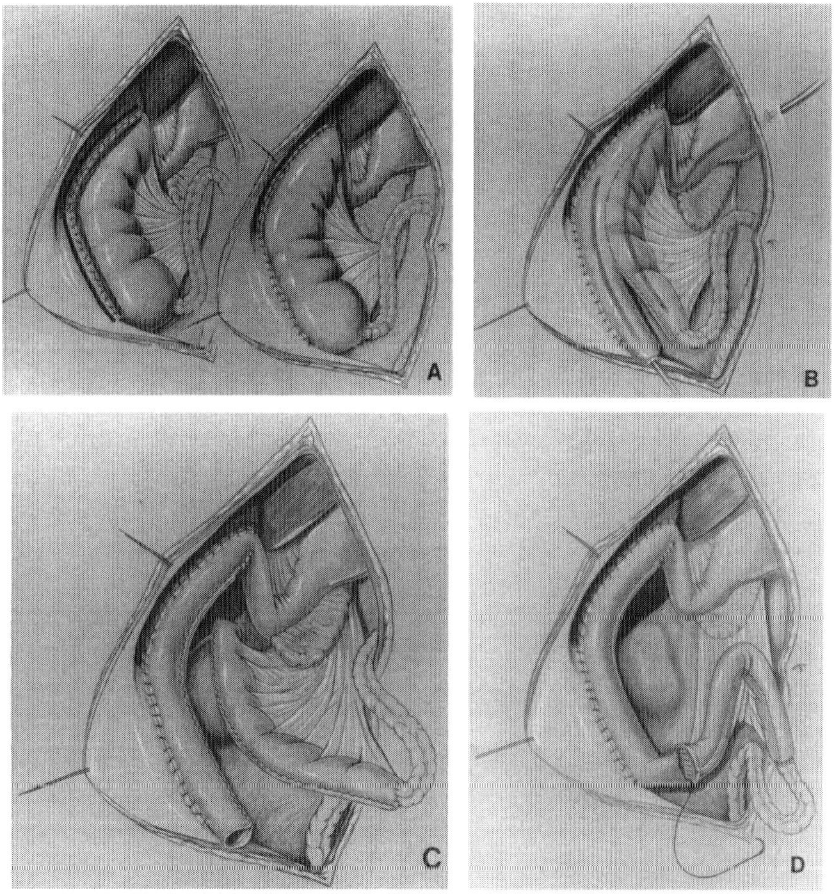

Figure 3. Original diagrams of the Kimura Technique [27]. A – Seromyotomy and coaptation of dilated small bowel to the liver. B – Longitudinal division of the dilated small bowel following collateral formation. C – Completion of division and mobilization of mesenteric portion. D – Anastomosis.

Current Techniques in Autologous Intestinal Reconstruction

The terms autologous intestinal reconstructive surgery (AIRS) and autologous gastrointestinal reconstruction (AGIR) emerged at the turn of the century to describe the collection of surgical techniques used in the treatment of SBS [30, 31]. By then, the two most commonly performed procedures were the LILT procedure, as described by Bianchi, and an emerging technique known as the serial transverse enteroplasty (STEP) procedure.

The LILT procedure, as described above, remained a popular procedure due to its effectiveness. While it underwent some minor alterations over the years, the major portions of the operation remained the same. Given its continued popularity, long term 20-year follow up data were recently published, demonstrating continued success in the management of the child with SBS [32].

Originally described by Kim et al. [33], the STEP procedure takes advantage of dilated bowel segments in SBS by performing alternating transverse divisions using a surgical stapler to create a "serpentine" bowel pattern (Figure 4). One of the key advantages to this method is the nearly doubling of intestinal length without the need of an anastomosis. Additionally, the procedure can be performed as a secondary procedure in patients who have previously had reconstruction [34-36]. Early follow-up data have been promising, demonstrating improved enteral tolerance and growth [37-39], but the procedure is not without drawbacks. As mentioned above, a repeat STEP procedure can be performed due to the fact that re-dilatation of the bowel following initial STEP is not an uncommon occurrence. The orientation of muscle fibers in the intestine following STEP is also a concern. The alteration of a uniform axis of muscular contraction has detrimental effects on peristalsis. It should be noted that peristalsis is often deficient in these patients as a sequela of their SBS, making it difficult to determine how impactful the procedure truly is on motility. Despite these drawbacks, the STEP procedure represents a significant advancement in the surgical management of SBS and one of the most common procedures performed today.

Experimental Techniques and Future Directions

Despite the success of the new era of intestinal lengthening, innovations continue with the goal of improved management of SBS. Progress is due in part to the fact that transplantation remains an option of last resort, improvements in immunosuppression and long-term outcomes notwithstanding.

The trophic effect of mechanical stress on tissues was initially popular in the orthopedic arena as it related to limb-lengthening [41, 42]. It wasn't until 1997 when Chen and later Printz applied the tension-stress principle to the lengthening of intestine. Using a rabbit model, the investigators showed that intestinal length could be increased via mechanical distraction, accomplished by an intraluminal tubular expander in the case of Chen and an extraluminal device in the case of Printz [43, 44]. Over the next several years, other investigators demonstrated the feasibility of mechanical distraction to induce "enterogenesis" in various animal models [45-47]. The most recent work in this area is taking advantage of next generation polymers and materials to design distraction devices which are easier to place and result in reliable lengthening [48, 49]. To date, these methods remain in the realm of animal models, although findings thus far are promising.

One of the more interesting techniques to emerge was the helicoidal enteromyotomy technique described by Dias et al. [50]. The impetus for its development was the fact that the LILT procedure required extensive handling of the mesentery and potential for disruption of blood supply as well as potential complications with multiple anastomoses. In a patient with short bowel these risks are especially significant. The procedure was theoretically advantageous because it provided bowel lengthening without opening of the lumen and, based on early data, without causing upstream dilatation. Subsequent studies have not been published to date, and thus helicoidal enteromyotomy remains in the very early stages of investigation.

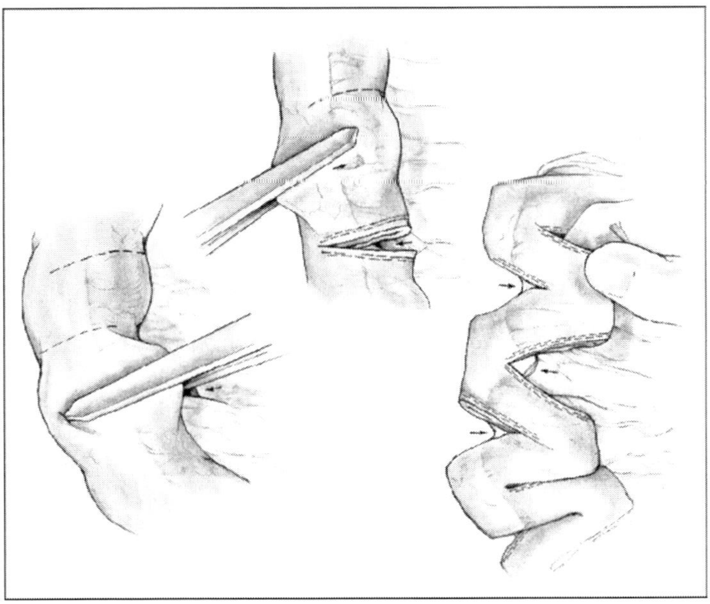

Figure 4. Serial Transverse Enteroplasty (STEP) procedure. Alternating subtotal transverse divisions of the bowel resulting in lengthening of a dilated segment [33].

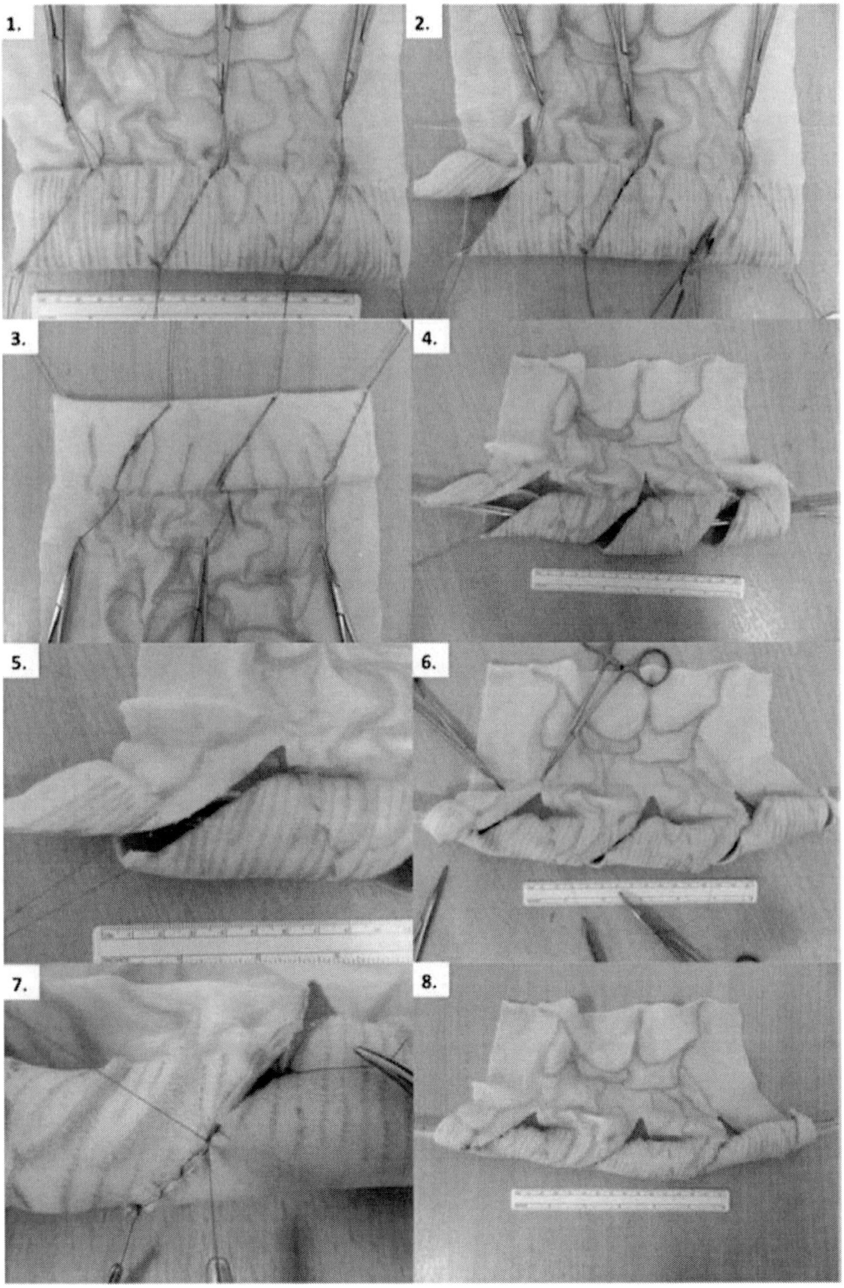

Figure 5. The SILT technique demonstrated on simulated bowel [52].

In a similar vein to helicoidal enteromyotomy, a group including Bianchi has recently developed a technique termed spiral intestinal lengthening and tailoring (SILT) [51]. Essentially a modification of LILT, this technique is based on the idea that a spiral segment of intestine can be "unwound" and then "rewound" such that the bowel is both longer and with a smaller caliber (Figure 5). Since its development, there have been a few clinical reports of the procedure in children with SBS [52, 53] with encouraging initial outcomes.

CONCLUSION

In the history of management of IF due to insufficient bowel length, surgery to improve the ability of the remaining bowel to meet the metabolic demands of the body has been an important and evolving component of care. From initial animal experiments to current AIR procedures, progress has been steady and rapid. The difficulty in management of the patient with IF due to SBS virtually guarantees the continued need for multimodal treatment. While difficult to predict the progress of intestinal transplantation, it is unlikely that alternative surgical treatments such as lengthening will ever become inconsequential. The current techniques have demonstrated value and emerging techniques hold promise in further advancement of this field and improvement in the daily lives of these patients.

REFERENCES

[1] Lowenfels AB. Intestinal Failure: Management Strategies. *ACS 2006 - Highlights of American College of Surgeons 92nd Annual Clinical Congress [Internet]*. 2006 11/5/2015. Available from: http://www.medscape.org/viewarticle/548912.

[2] Goulet O, Ruemmele F, Lacaille F, Colomb V. Irreversible intestinal failure. *Journal of pediatric gastroenterology and nutrition*. 2004;38(3): 250-69. PubMed PMID: 15076623.

[3] Howard L, Heaphey L, Fleming CR, Lininger L, Steiger E. Four years of North American registry home parenteral nutrition outcome data and their implications for patient management. *JPEN J. Parenter Enteral Nutr.* 1991;15(4):384-93. PubMed PMID: 1910101.

[4] Bines JE. Intestinal failure: A new era in clinical management. *J. Gastroenterol. Hepatol.* 2009;24 Suppl. 3:S86-92. doi: 10.1111/j.1440-1746.2009.06077.x. PubMed PMID: 19799705.

[5] Quiros-Tejeira RE, Ament ME, Reyen L, Herzog F, Merjanian M, Olivares-Serrano N, Vargas JH. Long-term parenteral nutritional support and intestinal adaptation in children with short bowel syndrome: a 25-year experience. *J. Pediatr.* 2004;145(2):157-63. doi: 10.1016/j.jpeds.2004.02.030. PubMed PMID: 15289760.

[6] Howard L, Ashley C. Management of complications in patients receiving home parenteral nutrition. *Gastroenterology*. 2003;124(6):1651-61. PubMed PMID: 12761723.

[7] Fishbein TM. Intestinal Transplantation. *New England Journal of Medicine*. 2009;361(10):998-1008. doi: doi:10.1056/NEJMra0804605. PubMed PMID: 19726774.

[8] Boluda ER. Pediatric small bowel transplantation. *Current opinion in organ transplantation*. 2015;20(5):550-6. Epub 2015/08/12. doi: 10.1097/mot.0000000000000231. PubMed PMID: 26262456.

[9] Singleton AO, Jr., Rowe EB. Peristalsis in reversed loops of bowel. *Ann. Surg*. 1954;139(6):853-7. PubMed PMID: 13159136; PMCID: PMC1609499.

[10] Gibson LD, Carter R, Hinshaw DB. Segmental reversal of small intestine after massive bowel resection. Successful case with follow-up examination. *JAMA*. 1962;182:952-4. PubMed PMID: 13947733.

[11] Warden MJ, Wesley JR. Small bowel reversal procedure for treatment of the "short gut" baby. *Journal of pediatric surgery*. 1978;13(3):321-3. PubMed PMID: 671198.

[12] Schiller WR, DiDio LJ, Anderson MC. Production of artificial sphincters. Ablation of the longitudinal layer of the intestine. *Arch. Surg*. 1967;95(3):436-42. PubMed PMID: 6035467.

[13] Waddell WR, Kern F, Jr., Halgrimson CG, Woodbury JJ. A simple jejunocolic "valve." For relief of rapid transit and the short bowel syndrome. *Arch. Surg*. 1970;100(4):438-44. PubMed PMID: 4906822.

[14] Lloyd DA. Colonic interposition between the jejunum and ileum after massive small bowel resection in rats. *Prog. Pediatr. Surg*. 1978;12:51-106. PubMed PMID: 704900.

[15] Glick PL, de Lorimier AA, Adzick NS, Harrison MR. Colon interposition: an adjuvant operation for short-gut syndrome. *Journal of pediatric surgery*. 1984;19(6):719-25. PubMed PMID: 6440966.

[16] Garcia VF, Templeton JM, Eichelberger MR, Koop CE, Vinograd I. Colon interposition for the short bowel syndrome. *Journal of pediatric surgery*. 1981;16(6):994-5. Epub. 1981/12/01. PubMed PMID: 7338785.

[17] Brolin RE. Colon interposition for extreme short bowel syndrome: a case report. *Surgery*. 1986;100(3):576-80. Epub. 1986/09/01. PubMed PMID: 3090727.

[18] Pressman A, Mogilner GJ, Siplovich L. [Interposition of colon for short bowel syndrome]. *Harefuah*. 1992;122(1):7-9. Epub. 1992/01/01. Pub Med PMID: 1551620.

[19] Bianchi A. Intestinal loop lengthening—A technique for increasing small intestinal length. *Journal of pediatric surgery*. 1980;15(2):145-51. doi: http://dx.doi.org/10.1016/S0022-3468(80)80005-4.

[20] Bianchi A. Intestinal lengthening: an experimental and clinical review. *J. R. Soc. Med.* 1984;77 Suppl. 3:35-41. PubMed PMID: 6471060; PMCI D: PMC1440516.

[21] Bianchi A. Longitudinal intestinal lengthening and tailoring: results in 20 children. *J. R. Soc. Med.* 1997;90(8):429-32. PubMed PMID: 930699 5; PMCID: PMC1296456.

[22] Chahine AA, Ricketts RR. A modification of the Bianchi intestinal lengthening procedure with a single anastomosis. *Journal of pediatric surgery*. 1998;33(8):1292-3. PubMed PMID: 9722007.

[23] Bianchi A. Experience with longitudinal intestinal lengthening and tailoring. *European journal of pediatric surgery: official journal of Austrian Association of Pediatric Surgery* [et al.] = Zeitschrift fur Kinderchirurgie. 1999;9(4):256-9. doi: 10.1055/s-2008-1072258. Pub Med PMID: 10532271.

[24] Weber TR. Isoperistaltic bowel lengthening for short bowel syndrome in children. *Am. J. Surg.* 1999;178(6):600-4. PubMed PMID: 10670880.

[25] Thompson JS, Pinch LW, Young R, Vanderhoof JA. Long-term outcome of intestinal lengthening. *Transplant. Proc.* 2000;32(6):1242-3. PubMed PMID: 10995930.

[26] Bueno J, Guiterrez J, Mazariegos GV, Abu-Elmagd K, Madariaga J, Ohwada S, Kocoshis S, Reyes J. Analysis of patients with longitudinal intestinal lengthening procedure referred for intestinal transplantation. *Journal of pediatric surgery*. 2001;36(1):178-83. PubMed PMID: 11150 461.

[27] Kimura K, Soper RT. A new bowel elongation technique for the short-bowel syndrome using the isolated bowel segment Iowa models. *Journal of pediatric surgery*. 1993;28(6):792-4. PubMed PMID: 8331504.

[28] Georgeson KE, Breaux CW, Jr. Outcome and intestinal adaptation in neonatal short-bowel syndrome. *Journal of pediatric surgery*. 1992;27 (3):344-8; discussion 8-50. Epub. 1992/03/11. PubMed PMID: 1501009.

[29] Georgeson K, Halpin D, Figueroa R, Vincente Y, Hardin W, Jr. Sequential intestinal lengthening procedures for refractory short bowel syndrome. *Journal of pediatric surgery*. 1994;29(2):316-20; discussion 20-1. Epub. 1994/02/01. PubMed PMID: 8176611.

[30] Jones BA, Hull MA, Kim HB. Autologous intestinal reconstruction surgery for intestinal failure management. *Current opinion in organ transplantation*. 2010;15(3):341-5. doi: 10.1097/MOT.0b013e328338c2 c0. PubMed PMID: 20386447.

[31] Bianchi A. From the cradle to enteral autonomy: the role of autologous gastrointestinal reconstruction. *Gastroenterology*. 2006;130(2 Suppl. 1): S138-46. doi: 10.1053/j.gastro.2005.09.070. PubMed PMID: 16473062.

[32] Walker SR, Nucci A, Yaworski JA, Barksdale EM, Jr. The Bianchi procedure: a 20-year single institution experience. *Journal of pediatric surgery*. 2006;41(1):113-9; discussion-9. doi: 10.1016/j.jpedsurg.2005. 10.015. PubMed PMID: 16410119.

[33] Kim HB, Fauza D, Garza J, Oh JT, Nurko S, Jaksic T. Serial transverse enteroplasty (STEP): a novel bowel lengthening procedure. *Journal of pediatric surgery*. 2003;38(3):425-9. doi: 10.1053/jpsu.2003.50073. Pub Med PMID: 12632361.

[34] Piper H, Modi BP, Kim HB, Fauza D, Glickman J, Jaksic T. The second STEP: the feasibility of repeat serial transverse enteroplasty. *Journal of pediatric surgery*. 2006;41(12):1951-6. doi: 10.1016/j.jpedsurg.2006.08. 015. PubMed PMID: 17161180.

[35] Andres AM, Thompson J, Grant W, Botha J, Sunderman B, Antonson D, Langnas A, Sudan D. Repeat surgical bowel lengthening with the STEP procedure. *Transplantation*. 2008;85(9):1294-9. doi: 10.1097/TP.0b013e 31817268ca. PubMed PMID: 18475187.

[36] Ehrlich PF, Mychaliska GB, Teitelbaum DH. The 2 STEP: an approach to repeating a serial transverse enteroplasty. *Journal of pediatric surgery*. 2007;42(5):819-22. doi: 10.1016/j.jpedsurg.2006.12.056. Pub Med PMID: 17502191.

[37] Garnett GM, Kang KH, Jaksic T, Woo RK, Puapong DP, Kim HB, Johnson SM. First STEPs: serial transverse enteroplasty as a primary procedure in neonates with congenital short bowel. *Journal of pediatric surgery*. 2014;49(1):104-7; discussion 8. Epub. 2014/01/21. doi: 10. 1016/j.jpedsurg.2013.09.037. PubMed PMID: 24439591.

[38] Oh PS, Fingeret AL, Shah MY, Ventura KA, Brodlie S, Ovchinsky N, Martinez M, Lobritto SJ, Cowles RA. Improved tolerance for enteral nutrition after serial transverse enteroplasty (STEP) in infants and children with short bowel syndrome--a seven-year single-center experience. *Journal of pediatric surgery*. 2014;49(11):1589-92. Epub 2014/12/06. doi: 10.1016/j.jpedsurg.2014.07.019. PubMed PMID: 2547 5799.

[39] Ching YA, Fitzgibbons S, Valim C, Zhou J, Duggan C, Jaksic T, Kim HB. Long-term nutritional and clinical outcomes after serial transverse enteroplasty at a single institution. *Journal of pediatric surgery*. 2009;44 (5):939-43. doi: 10.1016/j.jpedsurg.2009.01.070. PubMed PMID: 19433 174; PMCID: PMC3217836.

[40] Chang RW, Javid PJ, Oh JT, Andreoli S, Kim HB, Fauza D, Jaksic T. Serial transverse enteroplasty enhances intestinal function in a model of short bowel syndrome. *Ann. Surg*. 2006;243(2):223-8. doi: 10.1097/01. sla.0000197704.76166.07. PubMed PMID: 16432355; PMCID: PMC14 48911.

[41] Ilizarov GA. The tension-stress effect on the genesis and growth of tissues: Part II. The influence of the rate and frequency of distraction. *Clin. Orthop. Relat. Res*. 1989(239):263-85. PubMed PMID: 2912628.

[42] Ilizarov GA. Clinical application of the tension-stress effect for limb lengthening. *Clin. Orthop. Relat. Res*. 1990(250):8-26. PubMed PMID: 2403497.

[43] Chen Y, Zhang J, Qu R, Wang J, Xie Y. An animal experiment on short gut lengthening. *Chin. Med. J*. (Engl.). 1997;110(5):354-7. PubMed PMID: 9594302.

[44] Printz H, Schlenzka R, Requadt P, Tscherny M, Wagner AC, Eissele R, Rothmund M, Arnold R, Goke B. Small bowel lengthening by mechanical distraction. *Digestion*. 1997;58(3):240-8. PubMed PMID: 92 43119.

[45] Park J, Puapong DP, Wu BM, Atkinson JB, Dunn JC. Enterogenesis by mechanical lengthening: morphology and function of the lengthened small intestine. *Journal of pediatric surgery*. 2004;39(12):1823-7. Pu bMed PMID: 15616941.

[46] Safford SD, Freemerman AJ, Safford KM, Bentley R, Skinner MA. Longitudinal mechanical tension induces growth in the small bowel of juvenile rats. *Gut*. 2005;54(8):1085-90. doi: 10.1136/gut.2004.061481. PubMed PMID: 15840689; PMCID: PMC1774906.

[47] Okawada M, Maria HM, Teitelbaum DH. Distraction induced enterogenesis: a unique mouse model using polyethylene glycol. *The Journal of surgical research*. 2011;170(1):41-7. Epub. 2011/05/25. doi: 10.1016/j.jss.2011.03.041. PubMed PMID: 21605872; PMCID: Pmc3154514.

[48] Fisher JG, Sparks EA, Khan FA, Dionigi B, Wu H, Brazzo J, 3rd, Fauza D, Modi B, Safranski DL, Jaksic T. Extraluminal distraction enterogenesis using shape-memory polymer. *Journal of pediatric surgery*. 2015;50(6):938-42. Epub. 2015/03/31. doi: 10.1016/j.jpedsurg.2015.03.013. PubMed PMID: 25812443.

[49] Scott A, Sullins VF, Steinberger D, Rouch JD, Wagner JP, Chiang E, Lee SL, Wu BM, Dunn JC. Repeated mechanical lengthening of intestinal segments in a novel model. *Journal of pediatric surgery*. 2015; 50(6):954-7. Epub. 2015/03/31. doi: 10.1016/j.jpedsurg.2015.03.020. PubMed PMID: 25818320.

[50] Dias AI, Martins JL, Moriya EM, Seda Neto J. Helicoidal enteromyotomy in rats: an experimental model of intestinal lengthening. *Transplant. Proc.* 2004;36(4):1012-4. doi: 10.1016/j.transproceed.2004.03.051. PubMed PMID: 15194352.

[51] Cserni T, Varga G, Erces D, Kaszaki J, Boros M, Laszlo A, Murphy F, Foldvari A, Morabito A, Bianchi A, Rakoczy G. Spiral intestinal lengthening and tailoring - first *in vivo* study. *Journal of pediatric surgery*. 2013;48(9):1907-13. doi: 10.1016/j.jpedsurg.2013.01.048. PubMed PMID: 24074666.

[52] Cserni T, Biszku B, Guthy I, Dicso F, Szaloki L, Folaranmi S, Murphy F, Rakoczy G, Bianchi A, Morabito A. The first clinical application of the spiral intestinal lengthening and tailoring (silt) in extreme short bowel syndrome. *J. Gastrointest. Surg.* 2014;18(10):1852-7. doi: 10.1007/s11605-014-2577-2. PubMed PMID: 24957255.

[53] Alberti D, Boroni G, Giannotti G, Parolini F, Armellini A, Morabito A, Bianchi A. "Spiral intestinal lenghtening and tailoring (SILT)" for a child with severely short bowel. *Pediatr. Surg. Int.* 2014;30(11):1169-72. doi: 10.1007/s00383-014-3583-x. PubMed PMID: 25119303.

BIOGRAPHICAL SKETCHES

Robert Anthony Cowles, MD

eRA Commons User Name: COWLESR

Position title: Associate Professor of Surgery, Yale School of Medicine

Institution and location	Degree	Year conferred	Field of study
University of Pennsylvania, Philadelphia, PA, US	BA	1991	Biology/ Chemistry
Temple University School of Medicine, Phila, PA, US	MD	1995	Medicine
University of Michigan Medical Center, Ann Arbor, MI, US	Internship Resident	1995-1996	Surgery
Institution and location	Degree	Year conferred	Field of study
University of Michigan Medical Center, Ann Arbor, MI, US	Resident	1996-2002	General Surgery
Columbia University College of Physicians and Surgeons, New York, NY, US	Clinical Fellow	2002 2004	Pediatric Surgery

Positions and Honors

Positions:

2004-2012: Assistant Professor of Surgery, Division of Pediatric Surgery, College of Physicians and Surgeons, Columbia University; Assistant Attending Surgeon, Morgan Stanley Children's Hospital of New York-Presbyterian

2012-Present: Associate Professor of Surgery, Section of Pediatric Surgery, Yale School of Medicine, New Haven, CT

Honors:

1987-1989 Citizen's Scholarship Foundation of America Scholarship
1992 US Healthcare Foundation Scholarship
1993 William Goldman Foundation Scholarship
1994 John Cresswell Memorial Award – for best performance on medicine rotation
1994 Alpha Omega Alpha Honor Society

1995	Emanuel M. Weinberger Award – for excellence in gastroenterology
1995	Association for Academic Surgery Surgical Student Research Award
1997, 2001	Bronze Beeper Award for excellence in resident teaching
1998	American College of Surgeons Resident Research Scholarship (1998-2000)

Selected Publications

Chen JJ, Gershon AA, Li Z, Cowles RA, Gershon MD. Varicella zoster virus (VZV) infects and establishes latency in enteric neurons. *Journal of Neurovirology* 17(6):578-589, 2011.

Cowles RA, Lobritto S, Ventura KA, Harren PA, Gelbard R, Emond JC, Altman RP, Jan DM: Timing of liver transplantation in biliary atresia – Results in 71 children managed by a multidisciplinary team. *Journal of Pediatric Surgery* 43(9):1605-1609, 2008.

Cowles RA, Moyer CA, Sonnad SS, Simeone DM, Knol JA, Eckhauser FE, Mulholland, MW, Colletti LM: Doctor-patient communication in surgery: Attitudes and expectations of general surgery patients about the involvement and education of surgical residents. *Journal of the American College of Surgeons* 193(1):73-80, 2001.

Cowles, RA, Segura, BJ, Mulholland, MW: Stimulation of rat pancreatic exocrine secretion by cocaine- and amphetamine-regulated transcript peptide. *Regulatory Peptides* 99(1):61-68, 2001.

Cowles, RA, Segura, BJ, Mulholland MW: Cocaine- and amphetamine-regulated transcript stimulates pancreatic exocrine secretion. *Surgical Forum* 51:28-30, 2000.

Cowles RA, Segura BJ, Mulholland, MW. Regulation of carbachol-induced c-fos mRNA expression in AR42J cells by somatostatin receptor subtypes 1, 2, and 3. *Pancreas* 25(3):239-244, 2002.

Cowles, RA, Turner, DJ, Segura, BJ, Romanchuk, GL, Mulholland, MW: Somatostatin inhibits carbachol-induced immediate early gene expression. *Surgical Forum* 50:42-44, 1999.

Cowles RA, Ventura KA, Martinez M, Lobritto SJ, Harren PA, Brodlie S, Carroll J, Jan DM. Reversal of intestinal failure-associated liver disease in infants and children on parenteral nutrition: experience with 93 patients at a referral center for intestinal rehabilitation. *Journal of Pediatric Surgery* 45(1):84-88, 2010.

Gross ER, Gershon MD, Margolis KG, Gertsberg ZV, Cowles RA. Neuronal serotonin regulates growth of the intestinal mucosa in mice. *Gastroenterology* 143(2):408-417, 2012.

Merchant, NB, Cordero, JA, Dempsey, DT, Cowles, RA, Milner, RA, and Ritchie WP, Jr.: The effect of somatostatin on bile acid-induced gastric mucosal injury. *Surgical Forum* 44:157-160, 1993.

Rangel SJ, Calkins CM, Cowles RA, Barnhart DC, Arca MJ, Teitelbaum DH. Parenteral nutrition-associated cholestasis: an American Pediatric Surgical Association Outcomes and Clinical Trials Committee systematic review. *Journal of Pediatric Surgery* 47(1):225-240, 2012.

Ruiz MJ, Thatch KA, Fisher JC, Simpson LL, Cowles RA: Neonatal outcomes associated with intestinal abnormalities diagnosed by fetal ultrasound. *Journal of Pediatric Surgery* 44(1):71-75, 2009.

Segura BJ, Cowles RA, Mulholland MW: The enteric nervous system: calcium signaling in enteric glia. *Recent Res. Devel. Neurochem.* 4:1-19, 2001.

Segura, BJ, Leach, KC, Cowles, RA, Mulholland, MW: Sphingosine-1-phosphate, lysophosphatidic acid, and sphingosylphosphorylcholine induce c-fos mRNA expression in C6 glioma cells. *Surgical Forum* 51:49-51, 2000.

Segura BJ, Zhang W, Cowles RA, Xiao L, Lin TR, Logsdon C, Mulholland MW. Lysophosphatidic acid stimulates calcium transients in enteric glia. *Neuroscience* 123(3):687-93, 2004.

Segura BJ, Zhang W, Xiao L, Turner D, Cowles RA, Logsdon C, Mulholland MW. Sphingosine-1-phosphate mediates calcium signaling in guinea pig enteroglial cells. *Journal of Surgical Research* 116(1): 42-54, 2004.

Segura BJ, Xiao L, Cowles RA, Zhang, WZ, Logsdon, CD, Mulholland, MW: Lysophosphatidic acid signaling in the enteric nervous system. *Surgical Forum* 52:3-5, 2001.

Turner, DJ, Cowles, RA, Segura, BJ, Romanchuk, GL, Barnhart, DC, Mulholland, MW: Cholinergic intrapancreatic neurons induce Ca^{2+} signaling and early-response gene expression in pancreatic acinar cells. *Journal of Gastrointestinal Surgery* 4(5):475-480, 2000.

Turner, DJ, Cowles, RA, Segura, BJ, Romanchuk, GL, Leach KC, Zhang, WZ, Mulholland, MW: Neuronal induction of c-fos transcription in pancreatic acinar cells occurs through muscarinic type 1 and 3 receptor subtypes. *Surgical Forum* 50:41-42, 1999.

Turner DJ, Cowles RA, Segura BJ, Mulholland MW. Cholinergic stimulation of rat acinar cells increases c-fos and c-jun expression via a mitogen-activated protein kinase-dependent pathway. *Journal of Gastrointestinal Surgery* 5(6):661-672, 2001.

Turner, DJ, Segura, BJ, Cowles, RA, Zhang, WZ, Mulholland MW: Functional overlap of inositol trisphosphate- and cyclic ADP ribose-sensitive calcium stores in guinea pig myenteric neurons. *American Journal of Physiology* 281:G208-G215, 2001.

Zhang, WZ, Turner, DJ, Segura, BJ, Cowles, RA, Mulholland, MW: ATP induces c-fos expression in C6 glioma cells by activation of P_{2Y} receptors. *Journal of Surgical Research* 94(1):49-55, 2000.

Research Support

Completed:

Neuroendocrine Regulation of Pancreatic Exocrine Function - American College of Surgeons – Resident Research Scholarship, 07/01/1998-06/30/2000.

Research Training in Surgical Gastroenterology – NIH-T32KD07698 (PI: Michael W. Mulholland, MD, PhD), 07/01/1998-06/30/2000.

Remodeling of the Enteric Nervous System After Massive Small Bowel Resection – The Charles Edison Fund, 07/01/2004-06/30/2008.

Vincristine Induced Changes in Gastrointestinal Motility: Effects on the Enteric Nervous System – Start-up Grant, Department of Surgery, Columbia University College of Physicians and Surgeons, 10/08/2007-06/30/2008.

Vincristine and the Enteric Nervous System: Neurotoxic Effects – Start-up Grant, Department of Surgery, Columbia University College of Physicians and Surgeons, 10/1/2008-6/30/2009.

The role of Serotonin (5-HT) on intestinal epithelial homeostasis - Start-up Grant, Department of Surgery, Columbia University College of Physicians and Surgeons, 10/1/2009-6/30/2010.

Regulation of intestinal responses to surgical stress by enteric nervous system-associated neurotransmitters – Kenneth A. Forde Award, Department of Surgery, Columbia University College of Physicians and Surgeons, 10/1/2009-6/30/2010.

The role of serotonin signaling on intestinal stem cell population – Start-up Grant, Department of Surgery, Columbia University College of Physicians and Surgeons, 10/1/2010-6/30/2011.

The effect of enhanced serotonin activity on intestinal absorptive capacity – Start-up Grant, Department of Surgery, Columbia University College of Physicians and Surgeons, 10/1/2011-6/30/2012.

Serotonergic Regulation of Intestinal Mucosal Repair – Ohse Grant, Department of Surgery, Yale School of Medicine, $30,000 to 6/30/2014.

Studies on enteric neurogenesis and neuroplasticity - Ohse grant, Department of Surgery, Yale School of Medicine, $40,000 to 6/30/2015.

Current:

Research Funding – Recruitment – Department of Surgery, Yale School of Medicine, $375,000, January 2013 to June 2017.

Chasen J. Greig, MD

Position title: Research Fellow - Yale-New Haven Hospital, Section of Pediatric Surgery

Education/training:

Institution and location	Degree	Year conferred	Field of study
Point Loma Nazarene University, San Diego, CA, US	BS	05/2008	Biology-Chemistry
Temple University School of Medicine, Philadelphia, PA, US	MD	05/2013	Medicine
Baystate Medical Center/Tufts University School of Medicine Program, Springfield, MA, US	n/a	Current	General Surgery Residency
Yale-New Haven Hospital, New Haven, CT, US	n/a	Current	Pediatric Surgery Research Fellowship

Positions and Honors

Positions and Employment:

2006-2008 Teaching Assistant - Introduction to Chemistry, Point Loma Nazarene University, San Diego, CA

2007-2008 Research Associate - Department of Biology, Point Loma Nazarene University, San Diego, CA

2008-2009 Laboratory Technician/Inventory Manager - Ambry Genetics Corporation, Aliso Viejo, CA

2010-2012	Research Associate - Sol Sherry Thrombosis Research Center, Temple University School of Medicine, Philadelphia, PA
2013-2015	Class Representative - Residency Leadership Group, Baystate Medical Center, Springfield, MA

Professional Memberships:

2009-	Student/Resident Member: American Medical Association
2013-	Resident Member: American College of Surgeons
2014-	Resident Member: Massachusetts Chapter, American College of Surgeons

Honors:

2004-2008	Tri-Beta National Biological Honors Society
2004-2008	Biology Department Honors Scholarship, Point Loma Nazarene University, San Diego, CA
2006-2008	NAIA and GSAC Scholar Athlete, Academic All-American
2008	Graduate, Magna cum Laude, Point Loma Nazarene University, San Diego, CA
2009-2013	Conwell Medical Scholars Award, Temple University School of Medicine, Philadelphia, PA

Contribution to Science

My early experience in basic science research began as a summer internship during college in the Microbiology Department with my mentor, Dr. Michael McConnell. I was involved with the sequencing of the genome of a novel bacteriophage, given the temporary name PLS-4. The study of this organism began after an experiment was performed in which Salmonella anatum A1 bacteria already infected with bacteriophage epsilon 15 was exposed to PLS-4. Up to that point, there had been no documentation of bacteriophage co-infection, as epsilon 15 had been shown to cause a change in the LPS layer of the bacteria rendering it seemingly inaccessible to numerous other bacteriophage. Given this novel finding of co-infection, our lab sought to further characterize this phage. My role early in the project was sequencing the entire genome such that we could compare it to other phage genomes to assess for differences. I designed primers based on the genome of epsilon 15, which we suspected to be similar based on other experiments, and amplified overlapping segments which were sequenced and pieced together to determine the sequence. Based on this, we found that PLS-4 had a polymorphism in the gene encoding the tail fiber. Subsequent experiments involving the creation of a chimeric DNA sequence with this polymorphism being incorporated into the epsilon 15 virion to attempt to induce co-infection were ongoing when I completed my time in the lab. I am hopeful that the sequencing data will be included in a publication once the necessary follow-up experiments are completed.

During medical school, I was fortunate work in the Sol Sherry Thrombosis Research Center at Temple University School of Medicine under Dr. A. Koneti Rao. His lab was interested in platelet storage pool disorders and I became involved in a project looking for a novel mutation in a patient under the care of Dr. Rao. This patient had a phenotype consistent with Hermansky-Pudlak Syndrome or HPS. This is a rare disorder characterized by oculocutaneous albinism. My role included PCR amplification of the candidate genes for HPS followed by sequencing, and RT-PCR followed by PCR for generation of cDNA to assess for genetic errors related to transcription. I successfully sequenced a total of 5 candidate genes without finding the mutation to explain the phenotype. There was the discovery of a pseudogene which was expressed in this patient, which is a relatively rare event, but did not explain the phenotype. When I left Dr. Rao's lab, there were several more candidate genes planned to be sequenced. Once a mutation is found, the data documenting normal sequence will be important to present in a future publication as those genes contain most of the known mutations for this disorder.

In: Short Bowel Syndrome (SBS)
Editor: Violet Chapman

ISBN: 978-1-63484-944-9

Chapter 4

RELATED NOVA PUBLICATIONS

SHORT BOWEL SYNDROME*

I. Sukhotnik
Technion-Israel Institute of Technology, the Ruth and Bruce Rappaport Faculty of Medicine, Department of Pediatric Surgery and Pathology, Bnai Zion Medical Center, Haifa, Israel

Short bowel syndrome continues to be an important clinical problem due to its high mortality and morbidity as well as to its devastating socioeconomic effects. The etiology of short bowel syndrome, its pathophisiology, the cellular and molecular mechanisms of intestinal adaptation are reviewed. Most common complication of short bowel syndrome including intestinal failure associated liver disease and sepsis are outlined with strategies to reduce them. The medical management and nutritional support of a patient with short bowel syndrome is complex and requires a multidisciplinary approach with the surgeon, gastroenteroliogist, pharmacist and dietitian working together. A review of the pharmacologic substances and growth factors that have been studied experimentally and administered clinically for the management of short bowel syndrome is presented. The mechanisms of action of peptide growth factors in intestinal cell proliferation as well as the effects of these

* The full version of this chapter can be found in *Gastrointestinal Disorders: Symptoms, Treatment and Prevention*, edited by Marouane Battik and Nesrine Grimaldi, published by Nova Science Publishers, Inc, New York, 2012.

factors on intestinal re-growth in an animal model of short bowel syndrome are discussed. Surgical options to promote intestinal adaptation and intestinal lengthening are described. Such knowledge may allow us to exploit various factors that act as growth agents for the remaining bowel mucosa and suggest new therapeutic strategies to maintain gut integrity after massive bowel resection, eliminate the dependence on total parenteral nutrition, and avoid the need for intestinal transplantation.

Short Bowel Syndrome: Definition, Incidence, Historical Overview and Etiology*

I. Sukhotnik, MD
Department of Pediatric Surgery, Bnai Zion Medical Center,
Technion-Israel Institute of Technology,
The Ruth and Bruce Rappaport Faculty of Medicine, Haifa, Israel

Short bowel syndrome (SBS) is defined as a condition of malabsorption that is due to reduction of functional intestinal mass necessary for adequate digestion and absorption for nutrient, fluid and growth requirements. SBS typically follows resection of 50% or more of the small intestine and is associated with diarrhea, steatorrhea, dehydration, electrolyte disturbances, malabsorption and progressive malnutrition. SBS is a functional rather than anatomic entity and its definition may be based on the need for intervention: patients requiring parenteral nutrition support for more than 1 to 3 months after massive small bowel resection can be defined as having SBS. The incidence of TPN-dependent SBS patients is estimated between 2 and 3 per million per year, with the prevalence at approximately 4 per year per million. In pediatric populations, SBS occurs in newborns and infants suffering from necrotizing enterocolitis, intestinal atresias, long-segment Hirschsprung's disease and malrotation with volvulus requiring massive intestinal resection. In adults, extensive resection is related to mesenteric vascular accidents,

* The full version of this chapter can be found in *Short Bowel Syndrome in Children: Current Practice and Future Perspectives*, edited by Igor Sukhotnik, published by Nova Science Publishers, Inc, New York, 2013.

malignancy, radiation strictures, adhesive obstruction and Crohn's disease. Other etiologies include trauma, fistula, scleroderma, radiation enteritis and intestinal obstruction. SBS has significant morbidity and is potentially lethal especially when intestinal loss is extensive.

SHORT BOWEL SYNDROME: PATHOPHYSIOLOGY AND INTESTINAL ADAPTATION*

I. Sukhotnik, MD

Department of Pediatric Surgery, Bnai Zion Medical Center,
Laboratory of Intestinal Adaptation and Recovery,
Technion-Israel Institute of Technology,
The Ruth and Bruce Rappaport Faculty of Medicine, Haifa, Israel

The degree and extent of malabsorption and metabolic complications seen in short bowel syndrome (SBS) depends on the site of intestinal resection. When the jejunum is resected, a temporary reduction in absorption of most nutrients occurs. However, when a significant portion of jejunum is lost, intestinal adaptation of the ileum can compensate for many of the jejunal functions. Major Ileal resections can reduce absorption of fluid, electrolytes, bile acids, and vitamin B12. These functions cannot be taken over by the remaining jejunum. A number of mechanisms contribute to malabsorption after massive resection, including acid hypersecretion, hypergastrinemia, rapid intestinal transit, impaired residual bowel, loss of surface area, bacterial overgrowth in dilated segments of small bowel, and bile acid depletion. Diarrhea in patients with short bowel syndrome is due to a combination of increased secretions, increased motility, and osmotic stimulation of water secretion because of malabsorption of luminal contents. The combined loss of absorptive surface area and compromised enterohepatic circulation, decreased bile acid pool and decreased pancreatic lipase secretion results in steatorrhea and inefficient fat absorption.

---

* The full version of this chapter can be found in Short *Bowel Syndrome in Children: Current Practice and Future Perspectives*, edited by Igor Sukhotnik, published by Nova Science Publishers, Inc, New York, 2013.

Mortality and Morbidity of Short Bowel Syndrome*

A. G. Coran, MD, and I. Sukhotnik, MD
University of Michigan, Section of Pediatric Surgery,
Mott Children's Hospital, Ann Arbor,
MI and Technion-Israel Institute of Technology,
The Ruth and Bruce Rappaport Faculty of Medicine,
Dept of Pediatric Surgery and Pathology,
Bnai Zion Medical Center, Haifa, Israel

Short bowel syndrome (SBS) continues to be an important clinical problem due to its high mortality and morbidity as well as to its devastating socioeconomic effects. The medical management and nutritional support of a patient with SBS is complex and requires a multidisciplinary approach with the surgeon, gastroenteroliogist, pharmacist and dietitian working together. The common causes of death in this population have been related to sepsis or intestinal failure associated liver disease. The use of parenteral and enteral nutrition in our daily practice has dramatically improved the outcomes during the past three decades. More than 90% of infants and children now survive after extensive small bowel resection in the neonatal period. Effectively caring for SBS patients and their families is a complex task that is best carried out in a coordinated, multi-disciplinary setting. The benefits of a multi-disciplinary approach include the stream-lined diagnosis and treatment, strengthened communication with families and the care teams, amalgamation of expert care, a holistic approach to patients, consistent follow up and continuity of patient care.

* The full version of this chapter can be found in *Short Bowel Syndrome in Children: Current Practice and Future Perspectives*, edited by Igor Sukhotnik, published by Nova Science Publishers, Inc, New York, 2013.

Management of Short Bowel Syndrome*

Rima Sohotnik and Ori Segol, MD
Department of Gastroenterology, Carmel Medical Center,
Technion-Israel Institute of Technology,
The Ruth and Bruce Rappaport Faculty of Medicine, Haifa, Israel

Management of children after massive bowel resection is optimized by interdisciplinary coordination of parenteral and enteral nutrition support, medical management of associated complications, surgical lengthening procedures, and intestinal transplantation. Individual plans of care are developed based on the length and sites of remaining bowel, the degree of intestinal adaptation, and the patient's ability to adhere to the medication and dietary regimens. Although patients require parenteral nutrition and/or intravenous fluids in the immediate postresection period, diet and enteral nutrition should be reintroduced as soon as possible. Antisecretory and antidiarrheal medications are prescribed to slow intestinal transit times and optimize fluid and nutrient absorption. The purpose of this chapter is to discuss the newest methods of optimizing pediatric parenteral and enteral nutrition in patients with SBS while ensuring growth, promoting intestinal adaptation, and reducing associated complications.

* The full version of this chapter can be found in *Short Bowel Syndrome in Children: Current Practice and Future Perspectives*, edited by Igor Sukhotnik, published by Nova Science Publishers, Inc, New York, 2013.

BOWEL-PRESERVING SURGERY FOR SHORT BOWEL SYNDROME*

Yechiel Sweed*†, *MD

Department of Pediatric Surgery, Nahariya Medical Center, Nahariya and Faculty of Medicine in the Galilee, Bar Ilan University, Safed, Israel

Short Bowel Syndrome (SBS) results in loss of absorptive capacity in the gut, leading to malabsorption due to protein, energy, fluid and electrolyte loss and imbalance while on the enteral diet alone. Various non-surgical and surgical therapeutic options have emerged that have improved the survival outcome following SBS in both children and adults. An individualized complex, multi-disciplinary approach to medical and surgical rehabilitation is needed to provide an opportunity for enteral autonomy to be possible in a patient with SBS. Multiple surgical techniques are available to address the patient with SBS. The two most commonly applied techniques are those labeled as intestinal lengthening procedures. These include the LILT (Longitudinal Intestinal Lengthening) described by Bianchi and the more recent STEP (Serial Transverse Enteroplasty) described by Kim. These "lengthening" procedures correct bacterial overgrowth by correcting the dilatation and dysmotility, leading to improved absorption and a decreased need for bowel transplantation. The remnant bowel of the patient with SBS plays a very pivotal role in autologous gastrointestinal reconstruction (AGIR) surgery. Intestinal transplantation should be reserved for patients with failed AGIR or those who have no prospect for autologous enteral autonomy.

---

* The full version of this chapter can be found in *Short Bowel Syndrome in Children: Current Practice and Future Perspectives*, edited by Igor Sukhotnik, published by Nova Science Publishers, Inc, New York, 2013.

† Address correspondence to Sweed Y, MD: Dept of Pediatric Surgery, Nahariya Medical Center, Faculty of Medicine in the Galilee, Bar Ilan University, Safed, Israel. E-mail: yechiel.sweed@naharia.health.gov.il.

BIBLIOGRAPHY

Beyond the NICU: comprehensive care of the high-risk infant LCCN: 2014013204 Main title: Beyond the NICU: comprehensive care of the high-risk infant /edited by William F. Malcolm, MD, Associate Professor of Pediatrics, Director, Intermediate Level Nurseries, Division of Neonatal-Perinatal Medicine, Duke University Medical Center, Durham, North Carolina; consultants, Ricki F. Goldstein, MD, Professor of Pediatrics, Director, High-Risk Infant Follow-Up Program, Division of Neonatal-Perinatal Medicine, Duke University Medical Center, durham, North Carolina, Richard J. Martin, MD, Drusinsky-Fanaroff Chair in Neonatology, Professor of Pediatrics, Rainbow Babies and Children's Hospital, Case Western Reserve University, Cleveland, Ohio, Betty Vohr, MD, Professor of Pediatrics, Medical Director, Neonatal Follow-Up Program, Women and Infants Hospital, Alpert Medical School of Brown University, Providence, Rhode Island. Published/Produced: New York: McGraw-Hill Education, [2015] ©2015 Description: xxiv, 968 pages: illustrations (some color); 22 cm ISBN: 9780071748582 (paperback: alk. paper) 007174858X (paperback: alk. paper) LC classification: RJ254. B49 2015 Variant title: Beyond the neonatal intensive care unit Related names: Malcolm, William F. (William Ferris), 1969- editor. Summary: "Beyond the NICU: Comprehensive Care of the High-Risk Infant delivers practical, evidence-based strategies for the care of convalescing NICU graduates in both inpatient and outpatient settings. In four sections, the book covers common problems shared by high-risk infants, role of various care providers from parents to specialists and timely interventions of therapy, timing and execution of transitioning the infant from intensive to convalescent care and from hospital to home, the etiology of chronic conditions affecting high-risk infants, details of convalescent care, discharge planning, and follow-up care for pediatricians"-- Provided by publisher. Contents: Machine generated contents note: Section 1 Introduction -- 1 History of the NICU -- 2 Commonalities of High Risk Infants: They're not all Preemies -- 3 Provider roles -- 4 Parent roles/wishes -- 5 Transitions for the High Risk Infant -- 6 Essential Components of a Comprehensive Follow-up Clinic -- Section 2 Medical Care of the Preterm Infant -- 7 Respiratory conditions of the preterm infant -- 8 Apnea and bradycardia -- 9 Patent ductus arteriosus -- 10 Adrenal Insufficiency -- 11 Nutrition and growth -- 12 Breastfeeding in the NICU Graduate -- 13 Necrotizing enterocolitis and short bowel syndrome -- 14 Gastroesophageal reflux -- 15 Catch-up Growth and Failure to thrive -- 16 Hypertension in the NICU Graduate -- 17 Anemia of prematurity -- 18 Thrombosis and Hematological Issues in the NICU Graduate -- 19 Hyperbilirubinemia -- 20 Endocrinopathies of the Preterm Infant -- 21 Bone Health -- 22 IVH, PVL, hypdrocephalus -- 23 Retinopathy of prematurity and ophthalmologic issues -- 24 Cerebral Palsy -- 25 Autism Spectrum Disorder -- 26 Intrauterine growth restriction -- 27 Post-NICU Issues of Multiple Gestation -- 28 Late Preterm Infants -- 29 Surgical issues -- Section 3 Medical Care of the Term Infant -- 30 Pulmonary Hypertension -- 31 Congenital diaphragmatic hernia -- 32 Congenital heart disease -- 33 ECMO and post-ECMO care -- 34 Congenital Intestinal anomalies -- 35 Maternal and neonatal infections -- 36 Birth asphyxia and HIE -- 37 Neonatal abstinence syndrome -- 38 Neural tube defects -- 39 Neonatal seizures and Infantile spasms -- 40 Infant of a diabetic mother -- 41 Down Syndrome -- Section 4 Developmental Care of the High Risk Infant -- 42 Early developmental issues in the NICU -- 43 NICU environment -- 44 Gross motor development -- 45 Fine motor development -- 46 Speech and language development -- 47 Feeding Issues in the NICU

Graduate -- 48 Hearing Loss -- 49 Neurodevelopmental testing - - 50 Neurodevelopmental outcomes -- 51 Family centered care and social issues -- 52 Palliative care -- 53 Early Intervention Services -- 54 Resources for providers and parents -- Appendices -- App A Discharging the high-risk infant -- App B Equipment needs of the high risk infant -- App C Medications -- App D Tests/Procedures -- App E Telephone Triage -- App F Coding and Billing. Subjects: Infant, Premature, Diseases--therapy. Infant, Premature. Comprehensive Health Care. Infant, Newborn, Diseases--therapy. Intensive Care, Neonatal. Notes: Includes bibliographical references and index.

Clinical handbook of pediatric gastroenterology LCCN: 2014037654 Main title: Clinical handbook of pediatric gastroenterology /edited by Rosemary J. Pauley-Hunter, Lisa Philichi. Edition: Second edition. Published/Produced: [Omaha]: The Association of Pediatric Gastroenterology and Nutrition Nurses, 2015. Description: p.; cm. ISBN: 9781576264850 (pbk.: alk. paper) LC classification: RJ446 Related names: Pauley-Hunter, Rosemary J., editor. Philichi, Lisa., editor. Association of Pediatric Gastroenterology and Nutrition Nurses. Contents: Abdominal pain / Rosemary J. Pauley-Hunter, Daphne Pierce-Smith, and Robin Shannon -- Allergic Conditions of the Gastrointestinal Tract / Rosemary J. Pauley-Hunter -- Celiac Disease / Mary-Alice M. Tully -- Constipation and Encopresis / Lisa Philichi -- Cyclic Vomiting Syndrome / Adelina Ferraro McDuffie and Anne Wuerth -- Diarrhea / Patricia A. Bierly -- Failure to Thrive / Kimberly S. Jarczyk, Shari Huffman, and Kelli Bissell -- Gastroesophageal Reflux / Lisa Philichi -- Gastrointestinal Bleeding / Robin Shannon -- The A, B, and C of Hepatitis / Patricia Turner Inflammatory Bowel Disease / Susan N. Peck - - Liver Disease / Angela Tendick, Cheryl Calabro, and Kristin Peterson-Madden -- Obesity / Kathleen Milliken and Nancy Murray -- Pancreatitis / Elizabeth Goldberg and Clare Ceballos -- Short Bowel Syndrome / Rosemary J. Pauley-Hunter, Rebecca C. Ratcliff, and Elizabeth E. Gleghorn -- GI Transplant / Cindy R. Brown, Shari Huffman, Brandi Gerhardt, and Patricia Turner -- Diagnostic

Studies / Diane Kocovsky -- GI Medications / Kathleen M. Gura, Shari Huffman, Lisa Philichi, and Maureen Egan -- Nutrition / Laura E. Beerman -- Feeding Tubes / Karen Sherry, Lillian R. Sablan, Corrine L. Maurins, and Emmala Ryan Shonce -- Growth Charts and Body Composition Analysis / Kimberly S. Jarczyk. Subjects: Gastrointestinal Diseases. Child. Infant. Liver Diseases. Pancreatic Diseases. Notes: Includes bibliographical references and index.

Nutritional management of hospitalized small animals LCCN: 2015007221 Main title: Nutritional management of hospitalized small animals / edited by Daniel L. Chan. Published/Produced: Chichester, West Sussex; Ames, Iowa: John Wiley and Sons Inc., 2015. Description: p.; cm. ISBN: 9781444336474 (cloth) LC classification: SF95. N888 2015 Related names: Chan, Daniel L., 1973-, editor. Contents: Nutritional assessment / Kathryn E. Michel -- Estimating energy requirements / Daniel L. Chan -- Routes of nutritional support / Sally Perea -- Nasoesophageal feeding tubes / Isuru Gajanayake -- Esophagostomy feeding tubes / Laura Eirmann -- Gastrostomy feeding tubes / Isuru Gajanayake, Daniel L. Chan -- Esophagostomy feeding tubes / Laura Eirmann -- Minimally invasive placement of post-pyloric feeding tubes / Matthew W. Beal -- Tube feeding: diet selection and preparation / Iveta Becvarova -- Intravenous access for parenteral nutrition / Sophie Adamantos -- Parenteral nutrition / Daniel L. Chan and Lisa M. Freeman -- Pathophysiology and clinical approach to malnutrition / Jason W. Gagne and Joseph J. Wakshlag -- Appetite stimulants / Lisa P. Weeth -- Adverse food reactions / Cecilia Villaverde and Marta Hervera -- Nutritional management of short bowel syndrome / Daniel L. Chan -- Refeeding syndrome / Daniel L. Chan -- Feeding patients with gastrointestinal motility disorders / Karin Allenspach and Daniel L. Chan -- Immune modulating nutrients / Daniel L. Chan -- Nutritional management of superficial necrolytic dermatitis / Andrea V. Volk and Ross Bond -- Nutritional support in acute kidney injury / Denise A. Elliott -- Nutritional support in hepatic failure / Renee M. Streeter and Joseph J. Wakshlag -- Nutritional management of the septic patient / Daniel L. Chan -- Nutritional support during acute pancreatitis / Kristine B. Jensen and Daniel L. Chan -- Nutritional support in the mechanically ventilated small animal patient / Daniel L. Chan -- Nutritional support in exotic pet species / Jeleen A. Briscoe, La'Toya Latney, and Cailin R. Heinze. Subjects: Animal nutrition. Veterinary nursing. Animal feeding. Veterinary diet therapy. Animal Nutritional Physiological Phenomena. Nutritional Support--veterinary. Nutritional Requirements. Nutritional Status. Veterinary Medicine--methods. Notes: Includes bibliographical references and index. Additional formats: Online version: Nutritional management of hospitalized small animals Chichester, West Sussex; Ames, Iowa: John Wiley and Sons Inc., 2015 9781119052968 (DLC) 2015015939

Short bowel syndrome in children: current practice and future perspectives LCCN: 2013952581 Main title: Short bowel syndrome in children: current practice and future perspectives / [edited by] Igor Sukhotnik. Published/Produced: Hauppauge, NY: Nova Science Publishers, Inc., 2013. Description: pages cm ISBN: 9781629485188 (hardcover)

The 5-minute pediatric consult LCCN: 2012012664 Main title: The 5-minute pediatric consult / editor, M. William Schwartz; associate editors, Louis M. Bell, Jr. ... [et al.]; assistant editor, Charles I. Schwartz. Edition: 6th ed. Published/Created: Philadelphia: Wolters Kluwer/Lippincott Williams and Wilkins, c2012. Description: xxx, 1113 p.: ill.; 28 cm. ISBN: 9781451116564 (hardback: alk. paper) 145111656X (hardback: alk. paper) LC classification: RJ48. A15 2012 Variant title: Five-minute pediatric consult Related names: Schwartz, M. William, 1935- Summary: "The 5 Minute Pediatric Consult provides immediate, practical advice on problems seen in infants, children, and adolescents. More than 450 diseases and conditions are covered in the fast-access two-page outline format that makes The 5-Minute Consult Series titles so popular among busy clinicians. Other features include a Chief Complaints section addressing the workup and treatment of 50 signs and symptoms, plus a medication index, syndromes glossary, surgical glossary, laboratory values, and tables all for quick reference saving you time and helping to treat your patients more efficiently.In this sixth edition, the 5 Minute Pediatric Consult also offers free 30 day access to the 5minuteconsult Pediatric website -- a clinical decision support tool -- that can be accessed by the health care providers to address questions on-the-go via website or mobile.New Features: New topics for this edition include: Amenorrhea, Asberger Syndrome, Dental Trauma, Head banging, Mental Retardation, Narcolepsy, Obsessive Compulsive Disorder, Separation Anxiety and Social Anxiety Free 30 Day Access to the 5minuteconsult Pediatric Website Includes More than 450 diseases and conditions to support your patient care decisions Patient education handouts from AAP to help educate your patients Hundreds of Images from Chung's "Visual Diagnosis and Treatment in Pediatrics" and other reputable sources to provide you with quick visual guidance Immunization schedules and charts at your fingertips to save you time from searching Content is optimized for handheld devices so you have access to the content anytime, anywhere Updates to content made on a regular basis to keep you abreast of the latest content Visit 5minuteconsult.com and click on the "go to pediatric consult tab" to learn more about your free access and begin using today!"-- Provided by publisher. Contents: Abdominal Mass -- Abdominal migraine -- Abdominal pain -- Abnormal bleeding -- Acetaminophen poisoning -- Acne -- Acquired hypothyroidism -- Acute drug withdrawal -- Acute kidney injury -- Acute lymphoblastic leukemia -- Acute myeloid leukemia -- Adenovirus infection -- Alcohol (ethanol) intoxication -- Allergic child -- Alopecia (hair loss) -- Alpha-1-Antitrypsin defficiency -- Altitude illness -- Amblyopia -- Amebiasis -- Amenorrhea -- Anearobic infections -- Anaphylaxis -- Anemia of chronic disease (Anemia of inflammation) -- Anicryptococcal infections -- Ankylosing spondylitis -- Anomalous coronary artery -- Anorexia nervosa -- Anthrax -- Aplastic anemia -- Appendicitis -- Arthritis, Juvenile idiopathic (Rheumatoid) -- Ascaris lumbricoides -- Ascites -- Aspergillosis -- Asplenia/Hyposplenia -- Asthma -- Ataxia -- Atelectasis -- Atopic dermatitis -- Atrial septal defect -- Attention-Deficit/Hyperactivity disorder

(ADHD) -- Atypical Mycobacterial infections -- Autism/Pervasive developmental disorder (PDD) Spectrum -- Autoimmune hemolytic anemia -- Avascular (aseptic) necrosis of the femoral head (HIP) -- Babesiosis -- Back pain -- Barotitis -- Bell palsy -- Bezoars -- Biliary Atresia -- Blastomycosis -- Blepharitis -- Bone marrow and stem cell transplant -- Botulism -- Brain abscess -- Brain injury, Traumatic -- Brain tumor -- Branchial cleft malformations -- Breast Abscess -- Breastfeeding Breastfeeding Jaundice and breast milk jaundice -- Breath-holding spells -- Bronchiolitis (See also: Respiratory syncytial virus) -- Bronchopulmonary dysplasia (Chronic lung disease of prematurity) -- Bruising -- Bruxism -- Bulimia -- C 1 Esterase inhibitor deficiency -- Campylobacter infections -- Candidiasis -- Carbon monoxide poisoning -- Cardimyopathy -- Cataract -- Cat-scratch disease -- Cavernous Sinus Syndrome -- Cavernous transformation and portal vein obstruction -- Celiac disease -- Cellulitis -- Cerebral palsy -- Cervicitis -- Chancroid -- Chest Pain -- Chickenpox (Varicella, Herpes Zoster) -- Child abuse, Physical -- Chlamydial infections -- Cholelithiasis -- Cholera -- Chronic Diarrhea -- Chronic granulmatous disease -- Chronic hepatitis -- Chronic kidney disease -- Cirrhosis -- Cleft lip and palate -- Clubfoot -- Coarctation of aorta -- Coccidioidomycosis -- Colic -- Coma -- Common variable immunodeficiency -- Complement deficiency -- Concussion -- Congenital hepatic fibrosis -- Congenital hypothyroidism -- Congestive heart failure -- Conjunctivitis -- Constipation -- Contact Dermatitis -- Contraception -- Cor pulmonale Costochondritis -- Cough -- Crohn disease -- Croup -- Crying -- Cryptococcal infections -- Cryptorchidism -- Cryptosporidiosis -- Cushing Syndrome (Adrenal Excess) -- Cutaneous Larva Migrans -- Cyclospora -- Cystic fibrosis -- Cytomegalovirus infection -- 22q11.2 Deletion Syndrome (Digeorge Syndrome) -- Dental/Oral Pain and urgencies -- Dermatomyositis/ Polymyositis -- Developmental disabilities -- Developmental dysplasia of the hip -- Diabetes insipidus -- Diabetes mellitus -- Diabetic ketoacidosis -- Diaper rash -- Diaphragmatic hernia (Congenital) -- Diarrhea -- Diphtheria -- Diskitis --

Disorders of sex development -- Disseminated intravascular coagulation -- Down (Trisomy 21) Syndrome -- Drowning -- Dysfunctional uterine bleeding -- Dysmenorrhea -- Dyspnea -- Dysuria -- Earache -- Edema -- Ehrlichiosis and anaplasmosis -- Encephalitis -- Encopresis -- Endocarditis -- Enuresis -- Endocarditis -- Epiglottitis -- Epstein Barr virus (Infectious Mononucleosis -- Erythema multiforme -- Erythema Nodosum -- Ewing Sarcoma -- Exstrophy of the bladder, cloacal exstrophy, and epispadias -- Failure to thrive -- Feeding disorders -- Fetal alcohol syndrome -- Fever and petechiae -- Fever of unknown cause -- Floppy infant syndrome -- Food allergy -- Food poisoning or foodborne illness -- Fragile X syndrome -- Frostbite -- Functional diarrhea of infancy or toddLer's diarrhea -- Fungal skin infections (Dermatophyte infections, Candidiasis, and Tinea Versicolor) -- Gastritis -- Gastroesophageal reflux -- German measles (third disease, Rubella) -- Giardiasis -- Gingivitis -- Glaucoma-- congenital -- Glomerulonephritis -- Gluecose-6-phosphate dehydrogenase deficiency -- Goiter -- Gonococcal infections -- Graft versus host disease -- Graves disease -- Growth hormone deficiency -- Guillain-Barre syndrome -- Gynecomastia -- Hand, foot, and mouth disease -- Hantavirus -- Head banging -- Headache and migraine -- Heat stroke and related illness -- Hemangiomas and other vascular lesions -- Hematuria -- Hemolysis -- Hemolysis -- Hemolytic disease of the newborn -- Hemolytic uremic syndrome -- Hemophilia -- Hemoptysis -- Henoch-Schonlein purpura -- Hepatic failure -- Hepatomegaly -- Hereditary Angioedema -- Hereditary spherocytosis -- Heroin intoxication -- Herpes simplex virus -- Hiccups -- Hirschsprung disease -- Histiocytosis -- Histoplasmosis -- Hodgkin Lymphoma -- Human immunodeficiency virus infection -- Human papilloma virus -- Hydrocephalus -- Hydronephrosis -- Hyperimmunoglobulinemia E Syndrome -- Hyperinsulinism -- Hyperlipidemia -- Hypertention -- Hypogrammaglobulinemia -- Hypoparathyroidism -- Hypoplastic left heart syndrome -- Hypospadias -- Idiopathic intracranial hypertension (Pseudotumor cerebri) -- Idiopathic Thrombocytopenic purpura -- Immune deficiency -- Immunoglobulin a deficiency --

Imperforate anus -- Impetigo -- In Inappropriate antidiuretic hormone secretion -- Infantile spasms -- Influenza -- Inguinal hernia -- Intestinal obstruction -- Intoeing-tibial torsion -- Intracranial hemorrhage -- Intussusception -- Iron deficiency anemia -- Iron poisoning -- Irritable bowel syndrome -- Jaundice -- Kawasaki disease -- Knee pain, Anterior/Patellofemoral malalignment syndrome -- Lacrimal duct obstruction -- Lactos intolerance -- Lead poisoning -- Learning disabilities -- Luekocytosis -- Lice (Pediculosis) -- Lower GI bleeding -- Lupus erythematosus -- Lyme disease -- Lymphadenopathy -- Malabsorption -- Malaria -- Mammalian bites -- Mastoiditis -- Measles (Rubeola, first disease) -- Meckel diverticulum -- Mediastinal mass -- Megaloblastic anemia -- Meningitis -- Meningococcemia -- Mental retardation -- Mesenteric adenitis -- Metabolic diseases in hypoglycemic newborns -- Metabolic diseases in acidotic newborns -- Metabolic diseases in Hyperammonemic newborns -- Metabolic syndrome -- Methemoglobinemia -- Microcytic anemia -- Milia -- Milk protein intolerance -- Mumps/Parotitis -- Munchausen syndrome by proxy -- Muscular dystrophies -- Myasthenia gravis -- Myocarditis -- Narcolepsy -- Neck masses -- Necrotizing entercolitis -- Neonatal alloimmune thrombocytopenia -- Neonatal apnea -- Neonatal cholestasis -- Nephrotic syndrome -- Neural tube defects -- Neuroblastoma -- Neurofibromatosis -- Neutropenia -- Non-Hodgkin Lymphoma -- Nosebleeds (Epistaxis) -- Obesity -- Obsessive compulsive disorder -- Obstetric brachial plexus (ERB) palsy -- Omphalitis -- Osteogenesis imperfecta -- Osteosarcoma -- Osteomyelitis -- Otitis externa -- Otitis media -- Pallor -- Pancreatic Pseudocyst -- Pancreatitis -- Panhypopituitarism -- Parvovirus B 19 (Erythema Infectiosum, fifth disease) -- Patent ductus arteriosus -- Pelvic inflammatory disease (PID) -- Penile and foreskin problems -- Pericarditis -- Periodic breathing -- Periorbital cellulitis -- Perirectal abscess -- Peritonitis -- Peritonsillar abscess -- Persistent Pulmonary Hypertension of the newborn (PPHN) -- Perthes disease -- Pertussis -- Pharyngitis -- Photosensitivity -- Pinworms --

Plague -- Pleural effusion -- Pneumoystic Jiroveci (Previously known as Pneumocystic Carnii Pneumonis) -- Pneumonia-- Bacterial -- Pneumothorax -- Polyarteritis Nodosa -- Polycystic kidney disease -- Polycystic ovary syndrome -- Polycythemia -- Polyps, intestinal -- Porencephaly cortical dysplasia/neuronal migration disorders-malformations of cortical development -- Portal hypertension -- Posterior urethral valve -- Premature adrenarche -- Premature thelarche -- Premenstrual syndrome (PMS) -- Primary adrenal insufficiency -- Prion diseases (Transmissible spongiform encephalophathies) -- Probiotics -- Prolonged QT interval syndrome -- Protein-Energy malnutrition (Kwashiorkor) -- Proteinuria -- Prune belly syndrome -- Pruritus -- Psittacosis -- Psoriasis -- Pubertal delay -- Pulmonary embolism -- Pulmonary hypertension -- Purpura fulminans -- Pyelonephritis -- Pyloric stenosis -- Rabies -- Rectal prolapse -- Refractive error -- Renal artery stenosis -- Renal tubular acidosis -- Renal venous thrombosis -- Respiratory syncytial virus (RSV) -- Retinoblastoma -- Retropharyngeal abscess -- Reye Syndrome -- Rhabdomyolysis -- Rhabdomyosarcoma -- Rheumatic fever -- Rhinitis, Allergic -- Rickets -- Rickettsial disease -- Rocky Mountain Spotted Fever -- Roseola -- Rotavirus -- Salicylate poisoning (Aspirin) -- Salmonella infections -- Sarcoidosis -- Scabies -- Scarlet fever -- Scleroderma -- Scoliosis (Idiopathic) -- Seborrheic dermatitis -- Seizures-febrile -- Seizures, partial and generalized -- Separation anxiety disorder -- Sepsis -- Septic arthritis -- Serum Sickness -- Severe acute respiratory syndrome (SARS) -- Severe combined immunodeficiency -- Sexual abuse -- Sexual ambiguity -- Sexual precocity -- Short-bowel syndrome -- Short stature -- Sickle cell disease -- Sinusitis -- Sleep apnea--obstructive sleep apnea syndrome -- Slipped capital femoral epiphysis -- Smallpox (Variola virus) -- Snake and insect bites -- Social anxiety disorder -- Sore throat -- Speech delay -- Speech problems -- Spinal muscular atrophy -- Splenomegaly -- Staphylococcal scaled skin syndrome (SSSS) -- Status epilepticus -- Stevens-Johnson syndrome and toxic epidermal necrolysis -- Stomatitis -- Strabismus -- Strep infection: invasive Group A Ç-hemolytic streptococcus -- Stroke -- Stuttering -- Subdural hematoma -- Substance use disorders -- Sudden Infant Death Syndrome (SIDS) -- Suicide -- Superior Mesenteric Artery syndrome -- Superior Mesenteric artery syndrome -- Supraventricular tachycardia -- Sympathomimetic poisoning -- Syncope -- Synovitis--transient -- Syphilis -- Tapeworm -- Teething -- Tendonitis -- Teratoma -- Tenanus -- Tetralogy of Fallot -- Thalassemia -- Thoracic insufficiency syndrome -- Thrombosis -- Tick fever -- Tics -- Toxic alcohols -- Toxic Shock syndrome -- Toxoplasmosis -- Tracheitis -- Tracheoesophageal fistula and esophageal atresia -- Tracheomalacia/laryngomalacia -- Transfusion reaction -- Transient erythroblastopenia of childhood -- Transient Trachypnea of the Newborn (TTN) -- Transposition of the great arteries -- Transverse myelitis -- Trichinosis -- Tuberculosis -- Tuberous sclerosis complex -- Tularemia -- Ulcerative colitis -- Upper gastrointestional bleeding -- Ureteropelvic junction obstruction -- Urethral prolapse -- Urinary tract infection -- Urticaria -- Vaccine adverse events -- Vaginitis -- Vascular brain lesions (Congenial) -- Ventricular septal defect -- Ventricular tachycardia -- Vesicoureteral reflux -- Viral hepatitis -- Volvulus -- Vomiting -- Von Willebrand disease -- Warts -- Weight loss -- West Nile Virus (And other Arbovirus Encephalitis) -- Wheezing -- Wilms tumor -- Wilson disease -- Wiskott-Aldrich syndrome -- Yersinia enterocolitica. Subjects: Pediatrics--Handbooks, manuals, etc. Pediatrics. Pediatrics--Handbooks. Notes: Includes bibliographical references and index. Series: 5-minute consult series 5-minute consult.

The importance of nutrition as an integral part of disease management LCCN: 2015027767 Main title: The importance of nutrition as an integral part of disease management / editors, Rémy F. Meier, Liestal, Switzerland, B. Ravinder Reddy, Hyderabad, India, Peter B. Soeters, Maastricht, The Netherlands. Published/Produced: Basel, Switzerland; New York: Karger; Vevey, Switzerland: Nestlé Nutrition Institute, [2015] Description: xiv, 156 pages; 25 cm. ISBN: 9783318054989 (hard cover: alk. paper) LC classification: RM217. I58 2015 Related names: Meier, Rémy F., editor. Reddy, B. Ravinder, editor. Soeters, Peter B., editor. Nestlé Nutrition Institute, issuing body. Contents: Basics in clinical medical nutrition / Meier, R.F., Forbes, A. -- Macronutrient metabolism in starvation and stress / Soeters, P.B. -- Noncaloric benefits of carbohydrates / Reddy, B.R. -- Biological value of protein / Moore, D.R., Soeters, P.B. -- Enteral nutrition: whom, why, when, what, and where to feed? / Reddy, B.R. -- Management of the metabolic syndrome and the obese patient with metabolic disturbances: South Asian perspective / Misra, A., Bhardwaj, S. -- Nutritional issues in the short bowel syndrome: total parenteral nutrition, enteral nutrition and the role of transplantation / O'Keefe, S.J.D. -- Nutrition in cancer / Ravasco, P. -- Nutritional therapy for critically ill patients / Martindale, R.G., Warren, M., Diamond, S., Kiraly, L. -- Perioperative nutritional intervention: where are we? / Hoos, T., Warren, M., Martindale, R.G. -- Health economics in medical nutrition: an emerging science / Nuijten, M. -- Nutrition, frailty, cognitive frailty, and prevention of disabilities with aging / Vellas, B., Secher, M., Gillette, S. Subjects: Nutrition Therapy. Notes: Includes bibliographical references and index. Series: Nestlé Nutrition Institute workshop series, 1664-2147; vol. 82 Nestlé Nutrition Institute workshop series; v. 82. 1664-2147

INDEX

A

B

C

D

E

F

G

H

I

J

K

L

M

N

O

P

Q

R

S

T

U

V

W

Z